THE TONGUE

NOT ESSENTIAL TO SPEECH:

WITH ILLUSTRATIONS OF THE POWER OF SPEECH IN

THE AFRICAN CONFESSORS.

By THE HON. EDWARD TWISLETON.

"Pessima enim res est errorum Apotheosis."—BACON.

LONDON:
JOHN MURRAY, ALBEMARLE STREET.
1873.

The right of Translation is reserved.

LONDON:
PRINTED BY WILLIAM CLOWES AND SONS,
STAMFORD STREET AND CHARING CROSS.

CONTENTS.

	PAGE
I. INTRODUCTION	1
II. CIRCUMSTANCES PRECEDING THE MUTILATION OF THE TONGUES	15
III. MUTILATION OF THE TONGUES AT TIPASA	30
IV. MODERN CASES OF PERSONS WHO HAVE SPOKEN WITHOUT TONGUES, OR WITH MUTILATED TONGUES	47
1. The Saumur Case	51
2. The Case attested by Dr. Tulp	54
3. The Portuguese Case	58
4. The Case of Margaret Cutting	77
5. The Case attested by Sir John Malcolm	97
6. Case attested by Mr. Wood, British Consul at Tunis	100
7. Cases attested by Sir John M'Neill	105
8. Cases attested by Dr. Wolff	110
9. Cases attested by Mr. Dickson	114
10. Case of Mr. Rawlings	120
11. Case attested by Professor Syme	150
12. Cases attested by Sir James Paget	157
V. CONCLUSION	162

Contents.

		PAGE
APPENDIX A.	The Original Authorities for the History of the African Confessors	169
,, B.	Dr. Newman's Remarks on the Evidence	176
,, C.	French Protestant Martyrs..	180
,, D.	Extract from M. Roland's French Work ..	183
,, E.	The Original Statement of Dr. Tulp respecting Joannes the Dumb	185
,, F.	Report of M. Jussieu to the French Royal Academy of Sciences on the Portuguese Case	187
,, G.	Dr. Newman on Roman Catholic Miracles	196
,, H.	Nine Miracles specified by Dr. Newman ..	198
,, K.	Tillemont on the Eternal Punishment of Arians..	216
,, L.	Edict of Honorius. A.D. 414	218
,, M.	Edict of Huneric. A.D. 484	221

ERRATA.

Page 15, line 1, *for* "439," *read* "429."
,, 76, ,, 1, *for* "F," *read* "B."
,, 124, ,, 10, *for* "operation," *read* "instrument."
,, 144, ,, 15, *for* "l's," *read* "t's."
,, 198, ,, 16, *for* "on," *read* "in."
,, 206, ,, 29, and elsewhere, *for* "Bishop Ambrose," *read* "Archbishop Ambrose."
,, 205, ,, 3 from bottom, *for* "flagrârant," *read* "flagrârunt."

THE TONGUE NOT ESSENTIAL TO SPEECH.

I.

INTRODUCTION.

BETWEEN Roman Catholics and orthodox Protestants there has never been a difference of opinion as to the truth of the miracles recorded in the New Testament; for to both, that truth is guaranteed by belief in the inspiration or special authenticity of the writings wherein those miracles are set forth. But the case is far otherwise as to belief in any subsequent miracles. Among orthodox Protestants the belief in these has fluctuated according to diversities in schools of theology and thought, or the intelligence and temperament of individuals: till in the course of the last century it eventually became weaker and weaker in proportion to the increasing strictness of the requirements for the historical evidence of common facts. And at length, with some reservation for the fiery eruptions supposed to have prevented the rebuilding of the temple at Jerusalem in the reign of the Emperor Julian, it may safely be asserted that in England, forty years ago, the value of miracles not recorded in the Bible was sunk so low in general estimation that they were regarded by the great majority of Protestant laymen with various feelings of indifference, neglect, distrust, disbelief, or contempt. The Church of Rome, on the other hand, has always laid claim to a succession of miracles. The alleged fact of such miracles is sometimes boldly appealed to as the stamp and the proof of its supposed divine commission; and in accordance with such a pretension, numerous Roman Catholic churches on the Continent teem with votive offerings, such as were common in pagan temples of old, which attest the belief of worshippers that, through the intercession of saints or of the Virgin Mary, their diseases have been miraculously healed. The degree to which beliefs of this kind are widely spread and deeply rooted is clearly set forth in the following extract from one of Dr. Newman's writings, published in 1851, after he had joined the Church of Rome:—

"Certainly the Catholic Church from east to west, from north to south, is, according to our conceptions, hung with miracles. The store of relics is inexhaustible; and each particle of each has in it at least a dormant, perhaps an energetic virtue, of supernatural operation. At Rome there is the true cross, the crib of Bethlehem, and the chair of St. Peter; portions of the crown of thorns are kept at Paris; the holy coat is shown at Trèves; the winding-sheet at Turin; at Monza the iron crown is formed out of a nail of the cross; and another nail is claimed for the Duomo of Milan; and pieces of our Lady's habit are to be seen in the Escurial. The Agnus Dei, blest medals, the scapular, the cord of St. Francis, all are the mediums of divine manifestations and graces. Crucifixes have bowed the head to the suppliant, and Madonnas have bent their eyes on assembled crowds. St. Januarius's blood liquefies periodically at Naples, and St. Winifred's Well is the source of wonders even in an unbelieving country. Women are marked with sacred stigmata; blood has flowed on Fridays from the five wounds, and their heads are crowned with a circle of lacerations. Relics are ever touching the sick, the deceased, the wounded: sometimes with no result at all, sometimes with marked and undeniable efficacy. Who has not heard of the abundant favours gained by the intercession of the Blessed Virgin? and of the marvellous consequences which have attended the invocation of St. Anthony of Padua? These phenomena are sometimes reported of saints in their lifetime, as well as after death, especially if they were evangelists or martyrs. The wild beasts crouched before their victims in the Roman Amphitheatre; the axeman was unable to sever St. Cecilia's head from her body; and St. Peter elicited a spring of water for his jailor's baptism in the Mamertine. St. Francis Xavier turned salt-water into fresh for five hundred travellers; St. Raymond was transported over the sea on his cloak; St. Andrew shone brightly in the dark; Santa Scholastica gained by her prayers a pouring rain; St. Paul was fed by ravens; and St. Frances saw her guardian angel. I need not continue the catalogue. It is agreed on both sides: the two parties join issue over a fact—that fact is the claim of miracles on the part of the Catholic Church. It is the Protestants' charge, and it is our glory."[a]

While a direct antagonism, such as is here described, existed between Roman Catholics and English Protestants respecting ecclesiastical miracles, Dr. Newman, before he wrote the above passage, and at a time when he was still in communion with the Church of England, published separately in 1843 an essay on the miracles recorded in the ecclesiastical history of the early ages. In that essay he fully admitted that miracles posterior to the Apostolic age were, on the whole, very different in object, character, and evidence from those of Scripture on the whole; but he main-

---

[a] 'Lectures on the present position of Catholics in England.' London, 1851, p. 291.

Introduction. 5

tained, at the same time, that there was no age of miracles after which miracles ceased; that there had been at all times true miracles and false miracles, true accounts and false accounts, and that some of the post-apostolic miracles were true miracles. And in illustration of these views he specified nine miracles, which he mentioned consecutively in detail, with the evidence for each respectively.

Of these miracles perhaps the most important was the one exhibited in the African confessors, who possessed the gift of speech though their tongues were said to have been cut out from the roots by order of the Vandal Arian, Huneric. This is the only ecclesiastical miracle which seems seriously to have baffled the historian Gibbon, who stated the evidence for the facts with perfect fairness, but did not attempt to explain them, and he concluded his notice of the subject with the following words:—"This supernatural gift of the African confessors, who spoke without tongues, will command the assent of those, and of those only, who already believe that their language was pure and orthodox. But the stubborn mind of an infidel is guarded by secret, incurable suspicion; and the Arian or Socinian who has seriously rejected the doctrine of the Trinity, will not be shaken by the most plausible evidence of an Athanasian miracle." [b]

---

[b] 'Decline and Fall of the Roman Empire,' chap. xxxvii.

In opposition to this incredulity, Dr. Newman devoted about twelve octavo pages to establishing the certainty of the facts, and insisting on their significance as miraculous.^c In his remarks he laid stress on the variety of the witnesses, and on the consistency and unity of their testimony in all material points. As striking features in the miracle, he dwelt on its completeness, on its permanence, on the number of the persons who were the subjects of it, and on its carrying its full case with it to every beholder. It was the miracle with which he concluded his essay, and the arguments in its behalf were somewhat more elaborate than for any other of the miracles in which he expressed his belief.

In 1854, Dean Milman, in a supplemental note to the first volume of his 'History of Latin Christianity,' published an extract from Colonel Churchill's 'Lebanon,' in which it is stated of certain emirs who had been punished by the loss of their tongues, that "the tongues grew again sufficiently for the purposes of speech." As a matter of fact, it is now deemed certain by physiologists that human tongues are incapable of growth; but still, as Colonel Churchill was a resident in the Lebanon, his statement that the emirs had been able to speak after their tongues had been cut out deserved attention. At any rate, after the

---

^c See Appendix B.

Introduction. 7

publication of Dr. Newman's essay, Dean Milman seems to have been the only writer who suggested a natural physical explanation of the supposed miraculous phenomena under consideration.

In January 1857, in reading Sir John Malcolm's 'Sketches of Persia,' I met with a passage which seemed to have a bearing on the speech of the African confessors, and I at once communicated on the subject with Sir John M'Neill, formerly British Ambassador in Persia, and with the late Sir Benjamin Brodie. Subsequently in 1858,[d] on the strength of information which they had most readily and courteously supplied to me, I published a memorandum in 'Notes and Queries,' the object of which was to show, 1st, that the punishment inflicted on the African confessors did not really deprive them of the whole of their tongues, and, 2ndly, that amputation of a portion of the tongue is not necessarily incompatible with the power of speech. In connection with this subject I adduced evidence to show the general prevalence of a belief in Persia that the excision of the tip of the tongue disables the sufferer from speaking, but that the faculty of speech is to a useful extent restored by

---

[d] The documents contained in this Memorandum had been previously communicated to Dean Milman, who referred to them in the second edition of his 'History of Latin Christianity,' published in 1857.

cutting out the whole portion of the tongue which is loose in the mouth. The question as to the correctness of that belief was reserved for future investigation, as although there was some evidence in its favour, that evidence seemed to be inconclusive. But this point did not bear one way or other on the miraculousness of the speech of the confessors. For, so far from its having been alleged that they had been merely deprived of the tips of their tongues, it had been expressly asserted and insisted upon that their tongues had been cut out or torn out by the roots.

After the publication in 'Notes and Queries' of the above-mentioned memorandum, cases came to my knowledge in which persons had been able to speak, although, from disease, they had lost apparently the whole of their tongues. And in 1862 I conversed more than once with Mr. Robert Rawlings, a person who could speak intelligibly, although by a comparatively new mode of operation the whole body of his tongue had been removed with the aid of an incision made under his chin. Still, although I took pains that the case should be known to scientific inquirers, I was not careful to publish anything concerning it; especially as some of the highest living authorities on such a subject regarded the evidence already adduced as amply sufficient for the rejection of the miraculous element from the history of the confessors. In reference to Dr. Newman himself the question of such miraculousness seemed a point of very secondary importance. He had advanced far beyond a belief in the nine miracles of his essay, or in any other supposed miracles recorded in the ecclesiastical history of the early ages. By becoming a convert to the Church of Rome he had accepted as a doctrine the astonishing and constantly recurring invisible miracle of transubstantiation; and, as will be seen from a passage already quoted, he had thrown himself fervently into the Roman Catholic system of belief respecting other miracles. He had stated that he thought it impossible to withstand the evidence for the liquefaction of the blood of St. Januarius at Naples, and for the motion of the eyes of the pictures of the Madonna in the Roman States. Moreover, he had individually expressed his firm conviction that "saints in their lifetime had before now raised the dead to life, crossed the sea without vessels, multiplied grain and bread, cured incurable diseases, and stopped the operation of the laws of the universe in a multitude of ways."

Within the last year, however, I became aware that Dr. Newman had republished in 1870 the essay of 1843 on ecclesiastical miracles, which he had written, not for Roman Catholics, but for members of the Church of England. In a note to this essay (p. 391) he reprints a passage from one of his previous works, in which he had dealt with the memorandum in 'Notes and Queries' respecting the African confessors. In that passage he fully allows that the point of evidence brought in disparagement of the miracle is *primâ facie* of such cogency, that till it is proved to be irrelevant (Roman) Catholics are prevented from appealing to it for controversial purposes. But he states that he should not be honest if he professed to be simply converted to the belief that there was nothing miraculous in the case of the African confessors. He expresses a wish to be quite sure of the full appositeness of the recent evidence; stating that questions of fact cannot be disproved by analogies or presumptions, and that the inquiry must be made into the particular case in all its parts as it comes before us.

Under these circumstances I have deemed it right to publish in the following pages a detailed account of the case of Mr. Rawlings, and likewise to set forth in order other well-attested cases of a similar kind. If belief in the supposed miracle had been abandoned unreservedly, as having arisen from an ignorance, by no means dishonourable, of existing natural organic laws, there might have been no reason for taking further notice of the subject. But the case is altered when, on the high authority of Dr. Newman, the miracle, though withdrawn from controversy, is not withdrawn wholly from belief. It is somewhat as if Naaman the Syrian, by a compromise which would not have suited his purpose, had been told that he must not enter the temple of Rimmon for public worship, but that he might carry about with him under his garments a small image of his god. And if an error is silently deified in the secret recesses of many individual minds, the general result may be scarcely less pernicious than if in the hands of priests with gorgeous vestments, amidst strains of plaintive or triumphal music, the apotheosis of the error takes place in solemn cathedrals, before high altars, in the presence of awe-stricken kneeling multitudes.

My immediate object in this publication is simply to show that there is no sufficient reason for importing the miraculous element into the history of the African confessors. But, independently of this point, the cases adduced deserve attention on general grounds, as proving that the tongue is not essential to the faculty of intelligible speech. There is reason to believe that, except in the medical profession, this fact is not generally known even now to educated men; and thus to some readers these cases may have a value as adding to their stock of scientific knowledge.

In reference, moreover, to ecclesiastical miracles, the case of the African confessors is interesting from its being apparently the only one of the nine miracles, specified by Dr. Newman, which does not partially depend on merely indirect evidence. This is a fact of some importance when it is borne in mind that those miracles were selected by a writer of undeniable ability, who is equalled by few among living men as a consummate controversialist, and who is thoroughly well acquainted with the events of early ecclesiastical history. For there is thus a guarantee that the selection has been carefully made, and that no other miracles can be pointed out which are supported by still stronger testimony. If these nine are too weak to bear the light of a searching scrutiny, there is reasonable ground for inferring that none other of the post-apostolic miracles are more robust and convincing. Hence it will not, perhaps, be a matter of indifference if one of the nine turns out to be no miracle at all, and if among the remaining eight not one is supported throughout by the testimony of witnesses who write as to what they themselves perceived by their own senses.

With these introductory remarks, I proceed to the main object of this work in the following order:—

1st. I shall give a general sketch of the historical facts which preceded the mutilation of the tongues by order of Huneric. Those who require more details in English are referred to the 33rd and 37th chapters of Gibbon's history, which contain a mine of valuable information, and which may, for the most part, be thoroughly relied upon for facts, as distinguished from opinions. No scholar, however, who is interested in the subject, should omit to read the Latin history of the Vandal persecution by Victor Vitensis, with the commentary by Ruinart. Victor was a contemporary Numidian bishop, called Vitensis from his see, of which the precise original name and the exact situation are not known. He published his history within a few years after the persecution; and if he sometimes uses expressions scarcely within the bounds of episcopal decorum and Christian meekness—such as calling Huneric "Bestia illa"—(compare Matthew v. 44; 1 Peter ii. 20, iii. 9)—he will readily be pardoned on account of the grievous wrongs which he had witnessed, and in consideration of the vivid idea which he presents of the African ecclesiastical mind towards the close of the fifth century. Ruinart was a learned French Benedictine (b. 1657, d. 1709), who performed the task of editing Victor's history with the same thoroughness on a small scale, according to his knowledge and ideas, which was exhibited in the seventeenth century on a larger scale by many French writers —such as Bochart, Du Cange, and Tillemont.

2ndly. I shall relate the circumstances attending the actual mutilation of the tongues of the confessors; and I shall adduce evidence to show that they were able, notwithstanding, to speak intelligibly, and that their power of speech was deemed miraculous.

3rdly. I shall specify instances wherein the suspicion of a miracle does not arise, of persons who have spoken intelligibly, although their tongues had been mutilated, or even, although the whole body of the tongue had been destroyed by disease, or had been removed by amputation.

And in the Appendix[*] I propose to show that the power of speech in the confessors, notwithstanding the mutilation of their tongues, is the only one of the supposed nine miracles specified by Dr. Newman, which is attested throughout by direct evidence.

---

[*] See Appendix H.

II.

THE CIRCUMSTANCES WHICH PRECEDED THE MUTILATION OF THE TONGUES.

IN the year 439 Genseric, with 50,000 Vandals, crossed over from Spain into Africa, and in a few years made himself master of the seven provinces in the north of that country, which had long formed a part of the Roman empire. These provinces, which are at present comprised, under different rulers, in the Pashalik of Tunis, in French Algeria, and in Morocco as far as Tangier, are now inhabited mainly by Mohammedans—the result of the wonderful conquests of the Arabs in the seventh century. But at the time of the Vandal invasion, the civilized inhabitants consisted chiefly of the descendants of Roman colonists, who had early embraced Christianity, who had entered with zeal into theological controversies, and who had produced more eminent ecclesiastical writers than Italy itself.[*]

---

[*] See Dean Milman's 'History of Latin Christianity,' vol. i. chap. i. Ambrose was an Italian, but Tertullian, Cyprian, and Augustine were all Africans. Jerome was born on the confines of Dalmatia and Pannonia.

The immediate success of the Vandals was mainly owing to the disloyalty of the Roman general, Boniface, who was governor of the African provinces at the time of the invasion. The Roman empire of the West, to which Africa belonged, was at that period ruled by the Empress Placidia, in the name of her son, Valentinian III.; and Boniface had been fraudulently induced to believe that an order for his return to Italy, which he had received from Placidia, was intended as a certain forerunner of his disgrace and death. From mixed motives of resentment and of apprehension for his personal safety, he had then formed an alliance with the Vandals, of which one of the principal conditions was the settlement of those barbarians in Africa. This treachery, of which Boniface soon bitterly repented, opened Africa to the Vandals. And their progress was facilitated by the half-savage Moors of the mountains and the desert, to whom the Romans had been unable to communicate their laws, religion, or language.

Still the essential causes of the Vandal conquest were far more deeply seated. The primary cause is to be found in the decay of the old Roman military virtues. The poet Ennius, in a memorable line,[b] which

---

[b] See Augustinus, 'De Civ. Dei,' 11, 21, and 'Historiæ Augustæ Scriptores,' Avidius Cassius, chap. v. The Emperor Marcus Aurelius speaks of it as "versum a bono poetâ dictum et omnibus frequentatum."

Cicero had praised for its oracular brevity and truth, had pointed out the real foundation of Roman greatness:

"Moribus antiquis stat res Romana virisque."

The Emperor Marcus Aurelius had quoted the same line in reference to the duty of enforcing a more rigid discipline among the legions in Syria; and it ought to have been sternly present to every Roman mind when, in the reign of the Emperor Gratian, the degenerate Roman infantry were allowed to lay aside the use of defensive armour, and were thus, according to Vegetius,[c] slaughtered by the barbarians like sheep. But the manners and men of the antique Roman mould had almost entirely ceased to exist; and as yet no substitute for them had been found in the new beneficent religion which had supplanted the worship of the ancient gods. If, indeed, Christianity in the fourth and fifth centuries had been like that religion which inspired the Swedes of Gustavus Adolphus, or the English Ironsides of Cromwell, it might, perhaps, have been possible to repel the invaders. But unfortunately the form which Christianity actually assumed involved a deification of

---

[c] See Vegetius de Re Militari, i. 20. His words are, "Sic dum exercitium laboremque declinant, cum maximo dedecore trucidantur, ut pecudes."

celibacy and of the monastic life;[d] and an ideal of excellence was presented to the human mind, in which patriotism was now no longer an indispensable virtue. At a time when nothing could have saved the empire but intense patriotism, fruitful marriages, encouragement of the military spirit, and regular training of the whole male adult population to the use of arms, men with ardent natures withdrew from active life into convents and hermitages, in which the salvation of their own souls, and not the salvation of their country, became the centre of their thoughts. Others entered the sacerdotal order, and instead of concentrating their physical and mental powers on beating back the barbarians, they wasted their energies on church councils, and on barren, though ingenious, speculations concerning the attributes and mode of existence of the three persons of the Christian Trinity. In addition, however, to this source of national weakness, Africa was suffering from the persecuting spirit in which the Roman Government had acted towards a religious body called the Donatists. These schismatics, so named from Donatus, a Numidian bishop, had finally separated from the African catholics in

[d] "I cannot praise a fugitive and cloistered virtue, unexercised and unbreathed, that never sallies out and sees her adversary, but slinks out of the race where that immortal garland is to be run for, not without dust and heat."—*Milton.*

consequence of feuds which had taken their rise from the election of Cæcilianus as bishop of Carthage in 311. The election of Cæcilianus had been objected to, on some minor grounds, as null and void; but the main ground of objection to it was that his consecration had been performed by a bishop who was a "traditor"—that is to say, a person who, in the time of Diocletian's persecution, had, in obedience to the law, given up holy vessels and copies of the Holy Scriptures to the civil power. The schism which resulted from this election might not have been politically injurious to the empire if it had been dealt with on the same principles as those which the Roman State had formerly adopted towards the various forms of Polytheism, or which the British Government has acted on in our time towards the members of the Scotch Free Church, who seceded in

---

* The schism of the Free Church resembles the schism of the Donatists in two respects—1st, that the schism did not involve any difference in doctrine; and 2ndly, that the seceding minority was singularly formidable from its magnitude. According to Gibbon, the Donatist bishops at the Conference of Carthage amounted to 279; and they asserted that their whole number was not less than 400. The Catholics had 286 present, 120 were absent, and 64 of their bishoprics were vacant. In the schism of the Free Church, 203 retired from the General Assembly, and 474 ministers signed the Deed of Demission, by which they resigned all claims to their stipends. A few more were subsequently added to the

1843 from the Church of Scotland. But the superstitious idea had gradually infected Christianity that those who did not believe in particular dogmas, or who did not conform to what was called the Catholic Church, would be condemned by the Deity in a future life to eternal torments.[f] This unworthy conception of the Supreme Being, which would sink him lower in the scale of morality on account of cruelty than Baal, or Moloch, or any Roman Catholic inquisitor of Spain, not unnaturally led to persecution. Mercy towards an infidel, a heretic, or a schismatic, was regarded with plausible logic as a culpable weakness; for it was argued that the temporal punishment of a few might be the means of saving many from everlasting fire. In accordance with these principles, the Emperor Theodosius had proscribed the sacrifices and ceremonies of Paganism under penalty of death; he had expelled the Arian bishops and clergy from all churches in his dominions; and he had prohibited, under severe penalties, all meetings of Arians for the purposes of public worship. In like manner the Roman government of his son, Honorius, employed, with the approbation of St. Augustine, similar weapons of persecution against the Donatists in Africa. By a

---

list. See the Article *Presbyterianism* in the 'Encyclopædia Britannica.' The 'Annual Register' for the year of secession gave 835 as the total number of Parish Ministers who then remained in the Establishment.   [f] See Appendix K.

decree[g] which Honorius promulgated in A.D. 414, a Donatist or a heretic was rendered incapable of inheriting or bequeathing property, and a fine graduated in amount, according to the rank of the offender, was imposed on any one who attended a Donatist religious meeting. If the offence was repeated five times, the case was to be specially referred to the emperor for severer punishment. By the same edict, still heavier penalties were inflicted on the Donatist clergy. Donatist bishops and presbyters, and other Donatists of the sacerdotal order, were to be banished to the islands or other provinces, and anyone who harboured or concealed any one of them in Africa was liable to the confiscation of all his property. By these means some hundred Donatist bishops, and several thousand Donatist clergy, were reduced to beggary and exile, and many Donatists were induced to conform to the Catholic Church. But others remained steadily and openly hostile to their oppressors; and the existence of a discontented and disaffected population was an important element in facilitating the progress of the Vandals. Although the Vandals were Arians, while the Donatists were Athanasians, the Donatists would naturally think that they could scarcely be treated worse by the Arians on the ground of heresy than they had been treated by the Athanasians on the

---

[g] See Appendix L.

ground of schism. Moreover, up to the time of the Vandal invasion, the Arians, either from policy, or through the teachings of the admirable missionary Ulphilas, from whom they had received Christianity, had never systematically returned evil for evil by persecuting Athanasians. Hence the Donatists, attaching more weight to present certain evils than to future uncertain dangers, would be disposed, secretly or openly, to favour the Vandals.

Genseric lived forty-eight years after his landing in Africa. It was his singular destiny to capture both the renowned cities which had once been rivals for the dominion of western Europe. He took Carthage in 439, and occupied it as the capital of his empire. He took and plundered Rome in 455. The celebrated Augustine, bishop of Hippo Regius in Numidia, had died in 430 during the siege of that city by the Vandals; having just lived to see some of the calamities which his principles of persecution had contributed to bring on his native land. He had strenuously opposed putting Donatists to death; but he had approved of inflicting banishment and confiscation of property on the Donatist clergy, and in the examination of Donatists he had likewise sanctioned the infliction of flogging.[b] If he who was a Christian

---

[b] In a letter to Count Marcellinus, Augustine writes:—
"Noli perdere paternam diligentiam quam in ipsâ inquisitione

bishop, and who may be regarded as one of the highest products of Roman civilisation among the African Catholics went so far as this, it can scarcely be a matter for surprise that barbarians from the north did not confine their intolerance within precisely the same limits. Genseric oppressed and persecuted the Catholics in various ways, and in the use of torture was certainly not satisfied with the paternal punishment of flogging. Yet in the main outlines of his persecution he merely copied measures which had been adopted by Catholics against Arians. In parts of Africa Catholic conventicles were wholly prohibited, and during the last twenty-four years of his reign he would not allow the election of a Catholic bishop at Carthage. But religious persecution was not the dominant passion in his mind. He delighted in war and plunder, and, like many other conquerors, he was a terrible scourge to mankind! Indeed he may have half regarded himself as a scourge sent by God, if we may accept as serious his answer to his pilot, who asked him on leaving Carthage whither he was to

---

servasti, quando tantorum scelerum confessionem non sulcantibus ungulis, non urentibus flammis, sed virgarum verberibus eruisti; qui modus coercitionis et a magistris artium liberalium et ab ipsis parentibus adhibetur, et sæpe etiam in judiciis solet ab Episcopis adhiberi." See Epistle 132.—Vol. ii. p. 518, 'Augustini Opera,' edition of 1807.

steer, and was told in reply, "against those with whom God is angry."

Huneric, whose name is specially connected with the mutilation of the African confessors, succeeded his father Genseric as king of the Vandals in January 477, and died towards the end of 484, after a reign of seven years and ten months. Unlike his father, he seems to have been destitute of military ambition; but he was a man of savage cruelty, not sparing his own relations or even the priests of his own religious persuasion. Thus from motives of political suspicion he consigned Jocundus, an Arian bishop, to the flames, and he inflicted the same punishment on several Arian presbyters and deacons. But during the five or six first years of his reign, although with the approbation of the Catholics he persecuted the Manicheans, he did not persecute the Catholics themselves. Indeed, at the request of the Emperor Zeno and of Placidia, the widow of Olybrius, he permitted the Catholics to elect for themselves a bishop of Carthage, which naturally inspired them with cheerful hopes for the future.

These hopes did not last long. Whatever may have been his motives in granting that indulgence, Huneric seems afterwards to have determined to persecute Catholics with the same brutality which Philip II. manifested in later times in his endeavours to exterminate Protestants in his dominions.

He set about his task with an ingenious refinement of cruelty, by copying the mode of procedure which the Catholics, in the beginning of the fifth century, had adopted towards the Donatists. Before the final blow had fallen on the Donatists, the Emperor Honorius had caused a Conference to be held between them and the Donatists at Carthage. In like manner Huneric before issuing a final edict against the Catholics, determined that the same city should witness a Conference between the Catholics and the Arians. Accordingly on Ascension Day in June 483, he addressed an edict to Eugenius, bishop of Carthage, and to all other Catholic bishops in Africa, requiring them to be present at a Conference in Carthage on the kalends of February in the following year. The day arrived, and after postponement for a few days, the bishops assembled, 466 in number. This did not, however, take place until a bishop named, or rather misnamed, "Lætus," had been burnt alive, probably on the pretext of treason or some other political offence, but really for the purpose of intimidating the other bishops. The Arian bishop, Cyrila, was appointed to preside over the conference—a serious departure in point of form from the precedent of the conference between the Catholics and the Donatists, inasmuch as the Count Marcellinus, who had presided on that occasion, although an Athanasian, was at least a layman. On seeing Cyrila in the presidential chair, and hearing him called "patriarch" by the notary of Huneric, the Catholics remonstrated, and there was an uproar among them. For this offence all of them were ordered to be severely tunded or cudgelled,[1] but it is not specially stated that this corporal punishment was then actually inflicted. At any rate the Catholics had an opportunity to present their Profession of Faith. This document has some permanent importance as containing the earliest mention on record of the text respecting the Three Witnesses (1 John, v. 7), which though admitted into the New Testament in all the Bibles of modern Europe, is now allowed by the great majority of scholars to be spurious. This Profession of Faith is likewise interesting for its arguments respecting the Trinity, many of which would be admitted as sound in modern schools of Anglican divinity, though some are strangely fanciful, and founded on Latin mistranslations of the Old Testament. But whether the arguments in that document were sound or unsound was evidently immaterial. Huneric was prepared with an edict,[k] which, although it was not to become operative till June, he published in March.

---

[1] Victor's words are "Jubentur universi filii catholicæ Ecclesiæ qui aderant, centenis fustibus *tundi*," ii. 18. The words "tunded" and "tunding," which have long been used locally, deserve, perhaps, to be admitted into classical English. They might be used in cases wherein "beaten" and "beating" would be ambiguous.

[k] See Appendix M.

It is directed against the Catholics, called by him Homoousians. Its provisions are copied, as he asserts, from edicts issued by Catholics against those who were not of their own religious communion. He transcribes the penalties which they had imposed on heretics and schismatics; and, with a malicious pleasure which would have seemed to the Arians merely to breathe the spirit of righteous retribution, he proclaimed the enactment of precisely the same penalties against the Catholics. One law, edict, or provision which he transcribes as having been issued by Catholics, and which he retorts against them is especially worthy of notice; viz. that lax judges might be punished by proscription and death. This provision would be a terrible instrument in the hands of a tyrant to bend judges to his will; as they evidently would be in no danger from excess of severity, while they might at any time fall victims to the caprices of an unscrupulous ruler, if they were simply just and equitable, and unwilling to convict accused persons on insufficient evidence. This may tend to explain much that followed. For torture, which had always been sanctioned by the Roman law as a means of extracting truth from slaves, had often, under the later emperors, been illegally employed in ordinary causes against the free-born, and was positively legal, without any distinction between the slave and the free, in charges of treason. But spoken words, and not merely overt acts, would be regarded as treasonable; and it may be deemed certain that in a time of religious persecution many persons under the influence of religious zeal, would expose themselves to the charge of treason and become liable to torture, by angry curses, by devout prayers, and even by indiscreet casual words uttered against a cruel and heretical sovereign of a foreign race. With such formidable laws and pretexts at his command, Huneric soon commenced an atrocious persecution. In the language of Gibbon, "respectable citizens, noble matrons, and consecrated virgins were stripped naked and raised in the air by pulleys, with a weight suspended to their feet. In this painful attitude their naked bodies were torn with scourges, or burnt in the most tender parts with red-hot plates of iron. The amputation of the ears, the nose, the tongue, and the right hand was inflicted by the Arians." And, speaking of the Catholic bishops who had attended the Conference at Carthage, the same historian relates their fate as follows:—"One martyr and one confessor were selected among the Catholic bishops; twenty-eight escaped by flight and eighty-eight by conformity; forty-six were sent into Corsica to cut timber for the royal navy, and 302 were banished to different parts, exposed to the insults of their enemies, and carefully deprived of all the temporal and spiritual comforts of life."

Such was the state of things in North Africa, when Tipasa acquired celebrity as the scene of a barbarous punishment, and of an alleged miracle. I have deemed it right to mention numerous circumstances of an ancient date which preceded that punishment, because the atrocities perpetrated by Huneric on the Catholics are spoken of by Dr. Newman as "a suitable antecedent, and (if the word may be used) a justification of the miracle which followed." But the force of any such justification is much weakened by a knowledge of the principles on which Catholics had previously acted towards Pagans, Arians, and Donatists. The Catholics were responsible for that great corruption of Christianity which consisted in the persecution of those who did not believe in their dogmas, or belong to their religious communion. If for a while they suffered in an intensified form what they had inflicted on others, they still deserve that pity in great misery which is always due from man to man. But it would be unreasonable to regard them with any peculiar compassion, or to suppose that the cruel retaliation on them for their previous wickedness would form any special justification of a miracle.

III.

MUTILATION OF THE TONGUES AT TIPASA.

THE city of Tipasa, the scene of the supposed miracle, belonged to the Roman province of Mauritania Cæsariensis. Its ruins are still visible in a striking situation by the seaside, somewhat more than sixteen geographical miles to the west of the modern city of Algiers. In its vicinity is a picturesque mountain called the Chénoua, which at one point reaches the height of nearly 3000 feet, but which slopes down into a promontory, and forms a protection to the locality against westerly winds. At present the name of the city is merely preserved by an adjoining hamlet called *Tipàza*, which in 1866 had not more than 165 inhabitants, of whom 85 were French, 8 foreigners, and 72 natives. But ancient Tipasa was a city of some importance. It had been peopled in the first century by a colony of Roman veterans, and had received the right of Latium.[*] Its line of walls

---

[*] See Pliny, 'Nat. Hist.' vol. i.; and Joanne's 'Dictionnaire Géographique de la France,' under *Marengo*, in the supple-

Mutilation of the Tongues at Tipasa. 31

extended more than two miles in circumference; and ruins in it are still pointed out of a church about 196 feet long and 90 feet broad, of tanks for preserving water, of a theatre, a quay, a prætorium, and a gymnasium.

In order, as it alleged, to afford the Catholics time to be converted to the true religion, the edict of Huneric was not to take effect till the month of June. This gave the inhabitants of Tipasa opportunity for reflection and for concert as to the measures which they should adopt. They appear to have been peculiarly zealous Catholics, and when an Arian bishop was sent to take possession of the city as his see, they evidently regarded his advent with the same kind of abhorrence which was manifested by the Scotch Covenanters many centuries later at the intrusion into their churches of Episcopalian clergymen, or of the Anglican Liturgy. They had recourse to the desperate remedy of emigration. All who could find vessels embarked for Spain, and in this they were likely to be favoured by the season of the year, as in summer for several days, or even for several weeks together, the Mediterranean is sometimes as tranquil

---

ment. The ruins are not striking. M. Joanne states that the buildings have been used as a quarry by Arabs, Kabyles, Turks, and his own countrymen. Apart from historical associations, the principal interest of Tipasa is in the beauty of its situation.

as a lake, or is stirred only by gentle breezes. Very few of the inhabitants remained behind; and of these some deliberately braved the penalties of the edict by assembling for religious worship in one house publicly. For this illegality the offenders were punished by the amputation of their tongues and their right hands, and these are the persons known in ecclesiastical history by the name of the African confessors. The precise circumstances are related by Victor Vitensis, who is the sole trustworthy authority for details on this subject. After narrating other instances of persecution in Africa, he proceeds as follows:—"But let us hasten to make known, to the praise of God, what occurred at Tipasa, a city of the greater Mauritania. When the inhabitants saw that an Arian bishop had been appointed to their city by the notary of Cyrila for the destruction of their souls, all of them embarked on board ship and took refuge in Spain, leaving only a very few behind, who could find no vessels to carry them away. These last the Arian bishop endeavoured to convert to Arianism, at first by blandishments, and afterwards by the compulsion of threats. They, however, remaining strong in the Lord, not only laughed to scorn the madness of their adviser, but likewise, having assembled in one house, began to celebrate publickly the Divine mysteries. When this became known to the bishop, he secretly sent a report of their proceedings to Carthage. Huneric, on being informed of what had occurred, sent in anger a certain count to Tipasa, with a command that in the presence of the whole province he should cut off by the roots the tongues and right hands of the offenders in the middle of the Forum. The command was executed, but through the working of the Holy Ghost, they spoke and still speak just as they used to speak before. But if any one chooses to be incredulous, let him now repair to Constantinople, and there he will find one of them, the subdeacon Reparatus, conversing in polite discourse without any impediment. For which cause he is deemed peculiarly venerable, and the empress in particular regards him with the highest reverence."

It is to be observed that Victor Vitensis does not expressly assert in this passage that he himself had heard Reparatus, or any other of Huneric's victims converse after the mutilation of his tongue. In the case, however, of Reparatus at least, if not of the other confessors, this seems to be the most natural inference from his words, and such was evidently the impression which he intended to convey.

Independently of Victor's statement, there is other evidence on the same subject. This evidence is given fairly in a compressed form by the historian Gibbon; but it is presented more copiously in detail by Dr.

Newman. I propose to set it forth as it is presented by each of these eminent writers.

The following is Gibbon's statement of the evidence for the power of speech in the confessors, after mentioning the fact that their tongues had been amputated:—

"But the holy confessors continued to speak without tongues; and this miracle is attested by Victor, an African bishop, who published an history of the persecution within two years after the event: 'If anyone,' says Victor, 'should doubt of the truth, let him repair to Constantinople, and listen to the clear and perfect language of Restitutus, the sub-deacon, one of these glorious sufferers, who is now lodged in the palace of the Emperor Zeno, and is respected by the devout empress.' At Constantinople we are astonished to find a cool, a learned, and unexceptionable witness, without interest and without passion—Æneas of Gaza, a Platonic philosopher—has accurately described his own observations on the African sufferers: 'I saw them myself; I heard them speak. I diligently inquired by what means such an articulate voice could be formed without any organ of speech. I used my eyes to examine the report of my ears: I opened their mouth, and saw that the whole tongue had been completely torn away by the roots, an operation which the physicians generally supposed to be mortal.'[b] The testimony of Æneas of Gaza might be confirmed by the superfluous evidence of the Emperor Justinian, in a perpetual edict; of Count Marcellinus, in his chronicle of the times; and of Pope Gregory I., who had resided at Constantinople as the minister of the Roman pontiff. They all lived within the compass of a century, and they all appeal to their personal knowledge or the public notoriety for the truth of a miracle, which was repeated in several instances, displayed on the greatest theatre of the world, and submitted during a series of years to the calm examination of the senses."

In his notes to this passage, Gibbon gives some account of Æneas of Gaza; and in his references, mentions Procopius 'de bell. Vandal.,' c. i., c. 7, in addition to the other authorities quoted in his text He adds: "None of these witnesses have specified the number of the confessors. which is fixed at sixty in an old menology (*apud Ruinart*, p. 486)." He then refers to the two confessors who are said to have lost their tongues by dissoluteness; and he concludes with stating that "the miracle is enhanced by the

---

[b] It is remarkable that the words "an operation which the physicians generally suppose to be mortal," are translated by Gibbon from an interpolation in the Latin translation of Æneas, printed by Ruinart. In 'Notes and Queries,' of March 12 and April 16, 1859, I published some detailed remarks on this subject.

singular instance of a boy who had *never* spoken before his tongue was cut out "

The evidence as given by Dr. Newman is much more detailed, as it was part of his plan to cut off every loophole of escape from the conclusion that the African confessors were the subject of a miracle. This is useful for my own immediate object, which, in this branch of the subject, is mainly to present the evidence for the faculty of speech in the confessors, as fully as possible, as a fact, whether the fact was or was not miraculous. The fact itself has been presented in such a luminous manner by Dr. Newman that it would be a species of affectation to travel independently over precisely the same ground. At the same time his own words are valuable as showing with what strength of conviction, so late as 1843, he believed in the miraculousness of the fact which he proved. After several preliminary remarks, and after referring to the passage in Victor Vitensis, which I have already translated somewhat more fully, Dr. Newman translates[c] the evidence of six writers, viz. Æneas of Gaza, Procopius of Cæsarea, the Emperor Justinian, Count Marcellinus, Victor bishop of Tonno, and Pope Gregory I. Their evidence is set forth by him as follows :—

1. "Æneas of Gaza was the contemporary of Victor. When a Gentile, he had been a philosopher and a rheto-

---

[c] See Appendix A for the original passages.

rician, and did not altogether throw off his profession of Platonism when he became a Christian. He wrote a dialogue on the 'Immortality of the Soul and the Resurrection of the Body;' and in it, after giving various instances of miracles, he proceeds, in the character of Axitheus, to speak of the miracle of the African Confessors: 'Other such things have been and will be; but what took place the other day I suppose you have seen yourself. A bitter tyranny is oppressing the greater Africa, and humanity and orthodoxy have no influence over tyranny. Accordingly this tyrant takes offence at the piety of his subjects, and commands the priests to deny their glorious dogma. When they refuse, O the impiety! he cuts out that religious tongue, as Tereus in the fable. But the damsel wove the deed upon the robe, and divulged it by her skill when nature no longer gave her power to speak; they, on the other hand, needing neither robe nor skill, call upon Nature's Maker, who vouchsafes to them a new nature on the third day, not giving them another tongue, but the faculty to discourse without a tongue more plainly than before. I had thought it impossible for a piper to show his skill without his pipes, or harper to play his music without his harp; but now this novel sight forces me to change my mind, and to account nothing fixed that is seen, if it be God's will to alter it. I myself saw the men, and heard them speak; and wondering at the articulateness of the sound, I began to inquire what its organ was; and distrusting my ears, I committed the decision to my eyes, and opening their mouth, I perceived the tongue entirely gone from the roots; and astounded, I fell to wonder not how they could talk, but how they had "not died."' He saw them at Constantinople.

2. "Procopius of Cæsarea was secretary to Belisarius, whom he accompanied into Africa, Sicily, and Italy and to Constantinople, in the years between 527 and 542. By Belisarius he was employed in various political matters of great moment, and was at one time at the head of the commissariat and the fleet. He seems to have conformed to Christianity, but Cave observes, from his tone of writing, that he was no real believer in it, nay preferred the old Paganism, though he despised its rites and fables. He wrote the history of the Persian, Vandalic, and Gothic war, of which Gibbon speaks in the following terms: 'His facts are collected from the personal experience and free conversation of a soldier, a statesman, and a traveller; his style continually aspires, and often attains, to the merit of strength and elegance; his reflections, more especially in the speeches which he too frequently inserts, contain a rich fund of political knowledge, and the historian, excited by the generous ambition of pleasing and instructing posterity, appears to disdain the prejudices of the people and the flattery

of courts.' Such is Procopius, and thus he speaks on the subject of this stupendous miracle: 'Huneric became the most savage and iniquitous of men towards the African Christians. For forcing them to Arianize, whomever he found unwilling to comply, he burnt and otherwise put to death. And of many he cut out the tongue as low down as the throat, who even as late as my time were alive in Byzantium, and talked without any impediment, feeling no effects whatever of the punishment. But two of them having allowed themselves to hold converse with abandoned women, ceased to speak.'

3. " Our next witness, and of the same date, is the Emperor Justinian, who, in an edict addressed to Archelaus, Prætorian Prefect of Africa, on the subject of his office, after Belisarius had recovered the country to the Roman Empire, writes as follows : 'The present mercy which Almighty God has deigned to manifest through us for his praise and his Name's sake, exceeds all the wonderful works which have happened in the world—viz., that Africa should through us recover in so short a time its liberty, after being in captivity under the Vandals for ninety-five years, those enemies alike of soul and body. For such souls as could not sustain their various tortures and punishments by rebaptizing, they translated into their own misbelief; and the bodies of free men they subjected to the hardships of a barbaric yoke. Nay, the very churches sacred to

God did they defile with their deeds of misbelief; some they turned into stables. We have seen the venerable men who, when their tongues had been cut off at the roots, yet piteously recounted their pains. Others, after diverse tortures, were dispersed through diverse provinces, and ended their days in exile.'[d]

4. "Count Marcellinus, chancellor to Justinian before he came to the throne, is the fourth layman to whose testimony we are able to appeal. He, too, as two of the former, speaks as an eye witness, and the additional circumstances with which he commences seem to throw light upon Æneas's singular account, that the confessors spoke 'more plainly than before.' 'Through the whole of Africa,' he says, in his 'Chronicon,' under the date 484, 'the cruel persecution of Huneric, King of the Vandals, was inflicted upon our Catholics. For after the expulsion and dispersion of more than 334 bishops of the orthodox, and the shutting of their churches, the flocks of the faithful, afflicted by various punishments, consummated their blessed conflict. Then it was that the same King Huneric ordered the tongue to be cut out of a Catholic youth who from his birth had lived without speech at all; soon after he spoke, and gave glory to God with the first sounds of his voice. In short, I myself have seen at Byzantium a few out of the

---

[d] Cod. Just., lib. i., tit. 30, ed. 1553.

company of the faithful religious men, with their tongues cut off and their hands amputated, speaking with perfect voice.'

5. "Victor, bishop of Tonno, in Africa, Proconsularis, another contemporary, and a strenuous defender of the Tria Capitula, which were condemned in the Fifth Ecumenical Council, has left behind him a 'Chronicon' also, which at the same date runs as follows: 'Huneric, King of the Vandals, urging a furious persecution through the whole of Africa, banished to Tubunnæ, Macrinippi, and other parts of the desert, not only Catholic clerks of every order, but even monks and laymen, to the number of about four thousand, and makes confessors and martyrs, and cuts off the tongues of the confessors. As to which confessors, the royal city where their bodies lie attests that after their tongues were cut out they spoke perfectly even to the end. Then Lætus, bishop of the Church of Nepte, is crowned with martyrdom, &c.' It is observable from this statement that the miracle was recorded for the instruction of posterity at the place of their burial."

6. "Lastly, Pope Gregory I. thus speaks in his 'Dialogues': "In the time of Justinian[*] Augustus, when the Arian persecution raised by the Vandals

---

[*] This date is a mistake of St. Gregory's; also he calls them Bishops.—*Note of Dr. Newman.*

against the faith of Catholics was raging violently in Africa, some bishops, courageously persisting in the defence of the truth, were brought under notice; whom the King of the Vandals, failing to persuade to his belief with words and offers, thought he could break with torture. For when in the midst of their defence of the truth, he bade them be silent, but they would not bear the misbelief quietly, lest it might be interpreted as assent. Breaking out into rage, he had their tongues cut off from the roots. A wonderful thing, and known to many senior persons, for afterwards, even without tongue, they spoke for the defence of the truth, just as they had been accustomed before to speak by means of it. These then, being fugitives at that time, came to Constantinople. At the time, moreover, that I was myself sent to the emperor to conduct the business of the Church, I fell in with a certain senior, a bishop, who attested that he had seen their mouths speaking, though without tongues, so that with open mouths they cried out, 'Behold, and see; for we have not tongues and we speak.' And it appeared to those who inspected, as it was said, as if their tongues being cut off from the roots, there was a sort of open depth in their throat, and yet in that empty mouth the words were formed full and perfect. Of whom one, having fallen into licentiousness, was soon after deprived of the gift of miracle."

Dr. Newman then recapitulates the evidence as

follows:—" Little observation is necessary on evidence such as this. What is perhaps most striking in it, is the variety of the witnesses, both in their persons and the details of their testimony, together with the consistency and unity of that testimony in all material points. Out of the seven writers adduced, six are contemporaries; three, if not four, are eye witnesses of the miracle; one reports from an eye witness; and one testifies to a permanent record at the burial-place of the subjects of it. All seven were living, or had been staying at one or other of the two places which are mentioned as their abode. One is a pope, a second a Catholic bishop, a third a bishop of a schismatical party, a fourth an emperor, a fifth a soldier, a politician, and a suspected infidel, a sixth a statesman and courtier, a seventh a rhetorician and philosopher. 'He cut out the tongues by the roots,' says Victor, Bishop of Vite; 'I perceived the tongue entirely gone by the roots,' says Æneas; 'as low down as the throat,' says Procopius; 'at the roots,' say Justinian and St. Gregory. 'He spoke like an educated man without impediment,' says Victor of Vite; 'with articulateness,' says Æneas, 'better than before;' 'they talked without impediment,' says Procopius; 'speaking with perfect voice,' says Marcellinus; 'they spoke perfectly even to the end,' says the second Victor; 'the words were formed full and perfect,' says St. Gregory."

In closing this branch of the subject, it may be useful, as illustrating the treacherousness of memory, and the tendency to exaggerate in the narration of striking events, to call special attention to the mistakes made by Pope Gregory I. in the passage above quoted from his 'Dialogues.' Two of those mistakes have been very properly pointed out by Dr. Newman in a note, which I have reprinted, but it may be instructive to dwell somewhat on all of them. 1. Certain inhabitants of Tipasa, who had been unable to escape to Spain, assembled for purposes of public worship in the half-deserted city. These are spoken of by Pope Gregory as bishops, which palpably at once enhances the importance of what occurred. Yet there is no reason to believe that there was even a single bishop in the whole number. Under Huneric's edict every Catholic non-conforming bishop was liable to banishment; and if any such bishop had remained behind and braved the law, and been punished with the other confessors, it is improbable that Victor Vitensis, himself a bishop, would have failed to mention the fact. At any rate, even if there was one bishop among the confessors, it would be very misleading to describe them all as bishops. 2. Again, Huneric is represented as having broken into a passion because the confessors would not be silent at his bidding, in the midst of the defence of the truth. But Huneric had no personal relation with the confessors, when he gave the order for their punishment. He was not even present at Tipasa, but was residing at Carthage, five hundred miles distant. It seems certain, moreover, that the confessors were punished, not for persisting to argue when commanded to be silent, but simply for disobeying Huneric's edict against Catholic conventicles. Apart from the punishment of mutilation, which involves different considerations, the difference in the nature of the offence is important. The edict of Huneric merely proscribed Catholic conventicles, as imperial edicts had proscribed Arian and Donatist conventicles; and no impartial person would have felt any peculiar sympathy with the Catholics, if they had only suffered in adversity what, in the pride of prosperity, they had inflicted upon others. The case would have been different if Huneric had punished them in a fit of bad temper, because they had persisted in arguing when he had told them to be silent. The probable explanation of Pope Gregory's mistake is that he confounded in his memory the conference at Carthage with the occurrences at Tipasa. But this is merely a conjecture, and if it were correct, the fact would be only one of the many ways in which, through want of accuracy, erroneous statements are thrown into circulation. 3. A still more remarkable mistake of Pope Gregory I. is the anachronism into which he fell of supposing that Justinian was emperor when the tongues of the confessors were amputated. The truth is that Justinian at that time was not yet two years old, and he did not become emperor till more than forty-two years later, in April, 527. What renders this anachronism the more singular is that Gregory himself, according to his own statement, had once been at Constantinople on an ecclesiastical mission, and he might be supposed likely to have been well acquainted with the history of the African Vandals. At any rate it might be thought he could not have failed to know that there had been a wide interval of time between two such important ecclesiastical events as the persecution of the Catholics by the Vandal Huneric, and the accession of Justinian to the empire of the East,—especially as this last event preceded only by six years the total overthrow of the Vandal dominion in Africa.

These remarks are not made with any view of disparaging such an illustrious man as Pope Gregory I., better known as Gregory the Great, to whom Englishmen are indebted for the introduction of Christianity among their barbarian ancestors. But if even Gregory the Great was so inaccurate in the relation of historical facts, it is well to reflect how unsafe it would be to accept miraculous tales as true, solely on the hearsay evidence of inferior men, his ecclesiastical contemporaries, predecessors, or successors.

IV.

MODERN CASES OF PERSONS WHO HAVE SPOKEN WITHOUT TONGUES, OR WITH MUTILATED TONGUES.

IN the preceding section, evidence was adduced to show that the African confessors of 484 possessed the power of speech after their tongues had been amputated. From their time down to 1857, only one writer gave a correct explanation of the phenomenon, and with very few exceptions, all ecclesiastical writers, from Victor Vitensis to Dr. Newman, regarded the fact as miraculous. The object of this section is to set forth in order similar instances of the power of speech in which the hypothesis of a miracle is inadmissible.

In selecting these instances, care has been taken to exclude every case which rests solely on hearsay evidence. Hence, although there is contemporary evidence for the power of speech in some French Protestant Martyrs, who had to endure the mutilation of their tongues before they were burned alive at the time of the Reformation, yet as the fact of their speaking is not attested by any ear-witness or eye-witness, their case is not admitted into this section, but is transferred to the Appendix.[a]

I am aware of a few other cases in former times, and at the present day, dependent on hearsay evidence, or on merely indirect statements. Of these, some cases of the present day might, most probably, be substantiated by direct evidence, if carefully investigated and traced to original witnesses. But this may fairly be deemed superfluous, considering the strength of some of the cases recorded in this work.

For the knowledge of one very important case, viz., the one attested by Professor Syme (No. 11), I am mainly indebted to Mr. Fairlie Clarke, who has lately published a 'Treatise on the Diseases of the Tongue.' In that work he has mentioned, from a purely medical and scientific point of view, many of the cases set forth in this section. I especially desire, therefore, to call attention to what he has written on this subject.[b]

I have stated that previous to 1857 only one writer gave a correct explanation of the power of speech in the confessors. That writer was Dr.

---

[a] See Appendix C, p. 180.

[b] 'A Treatise on the Diseases of the Tongue,' by W. Fairlie Clarke, M.A. and M.B. (Oxon), F.R.C.S., Assistant Surgeon to Charing Cross Hospital. Renshaw, London, 1873.

Conyers Middleton, whose explanation will be found recorded at the close of the case of the Portuguese girl, which is the third case in the following series. Dr. Middleton, who was born in 1683 and died in 1750, is now chiefly known for his 'Life of Cicero,' which was first published in 1741. But he likewise published two works on ecclesiastical subjects; one in 1729, entitled 'A Letter from Rome, shewing an exact conformity between Popery and Paganism;' and the other in 1748, entitled 'A Free Inquiry into the Miraculous Powers which are supposed to have subsisted in the Christian Church from the earliest ages through several successive centuries.' It was in the last of these two works that he dealt with the case of the African confessors. His tone of thought and character of mind may to a certain extent be inferred from the titles of his works, and from the passage which contains his explanation of the supposed miracle. To this may reasonably be added the following passage, which is an extract from his preface to the 'Free Inquiry.'

"I persuade myself that the life and faculties of man, at the best but short and limited, cannot be employed more rationally or laudably than in the search of knowledge; and especially of that sort which relates to our duty, and conduces to our happiness. In these inquiries, therefore, whenever I perceive any glimmering of truth before, I readily pursue and endeavour to trace it to its source, without any reserve or caution of pushing the discovery of it too far, or opening too great a glare of it to the public. I look upon the discovery of anything which is true as a valuable acquisition to society, which cannot possibly hurt or obstruct the good effect of any other truth whatsoever: for they all partake of one common essence, and necessarily coincide with each other; and, like the drops of rain which fall separately into the river, mix themselves at once with the stream, and strengthen the general current."

Briefly, it may be said of him that, as a sincere lover of truth, he had an unappeasable hatred of Pious Frauds, in which, to use language not his own, "he saw the fraud, but did not see the piety." And he had a thorough conviction, based upon inquiry, that the claim to miracles on the part of the Church of Rome was the result of ignorance, mingled with imposture.

CASES.

1.—*The Saumur Case.*

The earliest case of speech without a tongue recorded by an eye-witness seems to be that of Pierre Durand, a French boy. This is attested by M. Jacques Roland, a surgeon of Saumur, in a special treatise on the case, which he published in that town in 1630. Nothing is now known of M. Roland except from his work. In its title page he is described as surgeon of Monseigneur the Prince (Gaston, Duke of Orleans, younger brother of Louis XIII.) and lieutenant of the first barber-surgeon of the king. He dedicates his work to a person somewhat better known, viz., Mr. Marc Duncan, a Doctor in the Faculty of Medicine, Professor of Greek, and Principal of the Academy of Saumur. Dr. Duncan (d. 1640) was a Scotchman who had married a Frenchwoman; and although named physician in ordinary to James I., he, for his wife's sake, declined to leave the country of his adoption. He is stated by M. Roland in the dedication to be the cause of the work, by having been the first person who called M. Roland's attention to the case. According to the fashion of the time, the volume contains many laudatory verses both in Latin and in French. Among them are six Latin verses and a French sonnet, written by Dr. Duncan's son ; in addition to another French sonnet and thirty-six Latin lines, written by an author named Du Maurier. These facts are mentioned merely to shew that the case had attracted general attention at Saumur.

The treatise is in seventy-nine pages of small octavo, and is entitled 'Aglossostomography, or description of a mouth without a tongue, which performs naturally all its other functions ;'[a] and, perhaps, Dr. Duncan is responsible for coining from Greek the long word of the title, which is well adapted to terrify any ordinary reader. The work is divided into seven chapters. Of these I reprint in the Appendix the first chapter, and the headings of the other chapters in the original French.

The statement of M. Roland respecting Pierre Durand is, that he was a boy between eight and nine years old, son of André Durand and Margaret Salé,

---

[a] The title in the original is 'Aglossostomographie, ou description d'une bouche sans langue, laquelle parle et fait naturellement toutes ses autres fonctions ; par M. Jacques Roland, Sr de Belebal, Chirurgien de Monsigneur le Prince, commis de son premier Médecin, et Juré à Saumur. A Saumur, pour Claude Gerard et Daniel de l'Erpinère. MDCXXX.'

labourers of the village of La Rangezière, in the parish of St. George, near Montaign, in Lower Poitou, who had fallen ill of the smallpox when he was between five and six years of age, and had lost the whole of his tongue by gangrene and mortification. "He spit it out," M. Roland writes, "bit by bit, without any vestige of it remaining. This, nevertheless, prevents him but very slightly from performing the five ordinary functions attributed to the part which he has thus lost. These, as we shall mention elsewhere, are the functions of speaking, of tasting, of spitting, of collecting food in the mouth, and of swallowing what is there. For this mouth without a tongue has newly acquired another conformation well adapted to these five actions, in order to supply the needs of the tongue, by the admirable considerateness of nature, which never omits opportunities of letting itself be seen as a mother to her children." M. Roland subsequently endeavours to explain, although not very satisfactorily, in the fifth chapter, how it is possible for a mouth to speak without a tongue.

The treatise of M. Roland cannot easily be procured in the original French; but in 1672, a Latin translation of it with notes, was published in the third volume of the 'Ephemerides Germanicæ,'[b] by

---

[b] The exact title of the work is as follows: 'Miscellanea Curiosa Medico-Physica Academiæ Naturæ Curiosorum,

Dr. Rayger, an eminent physician of Pressburg. The case of Pierre Durand thus became generally known to anatomists; as the 'Ephemerides Germanicæ,' commenced in 1670, were for Germany and for all scientific men who could read Latin, somewhat analogous to the 'Transactions of the Royal Society' of England, which had been commenced in 1665.

2.—*The case of Joannes the Dumb, attested by Dr. Tulp.*

About twenty-two years after the publication of the Saumur case by M. Roland, Dr. Nicolas Tulp, of Amsterdam, published an account of his having conversed with a man from whom all the loose part of his tongue had been cut out. Dr. Tulp (b. 1593, d. 1674)[c] was a person of note in his native land, and was distinguished by his civic virtues. He was four

---

sive Ephemeridum Medico-Physicarum Germanicarum Annus Tertius, Anni scilicet MDCLXXII, continens celeberrimorum Virorum tum Medicorum tum aliorum Eruditorum in Germania, et extra eam Observationes Medicas, Physicas, Chymicas, necnon Mathematicas, &c. &c. Lipsiæ et Francofurti, &c. Anno MDCLXXII.'

[c] There is a portrait and detailed biography of Dr. Tulp, S. V., in Kok's 'Vaderlandsch Woordenboek.' Amsterdam. 1793. He was father-in-law of the "Burgomaster Six" of Rembrandt.

times burgomaster of Amsterdam, and when he was seventy-nine years of age he contributed to resist the pusillanimous counsels of those who would have surrendered his native city to Louis XIV. But it was in medicine that he attained the greatest eminence. In the celebrated picture of Rembrandt, called "the Lesson in Anatomy," which is now at the Hague, Dr. Tulp, thirty-five years of age, is the professor who is giving the lesson, and who holds the dissecting knife over the dead body. And, generally, it may be said of him that he practised medicine with honour at Amsterdam during a period of half a century. The case of the man with the mutilated tongue is mentioned by him in a Latin work, called 'Observationes Medicæ,' which he published at Amsterdam in 1652. The circumstances of the case were the following.

A man called Joannes the Dumb, resided at Weesp, a small town eight miles south-east of Amsterdam. Joannes had become afflicted with the loss of speech through strange chances in life. In a voyage to Italy, he had fallen into the hands of Turkish pirates, who tried to make him embrace the Mahomedan religion. On his refusal to do this, they endeavoured to cut out his tongue by the roots through a wound under his chin; but failing in that attempt, they satisfied themselves with cutting out all the loose part of his tongue through the open mouth. The final result was that he became unable to speak. Three years afterwards, however, in Holland, he recovered his voice during a tempestuous night, after a shock of alarm from an unexpected flash of lightning. This occasioned great astonishment in his house and in the neighbourhood, and as rumours of the occurrence were noised abroad, they reached the ears of Dr. Tulp, who was induced to go to Weesp, to have an interview with Joannes.

Dr. Tulp's testimony is explicit as to the fact that Joannes had lost a great part of his tongue, and yet could speak. The following are his words :—

"The man who had been dumb during three whole years owing to the mutilation of half his tongue, him we heard, with the same defect, not only distinctly speaking, but likewise pronouncing accurately one and all the consonants, the enunciation of which is attributed by the most sagacious investigators of Nature to the tip of the tongue alone.

"For speech is not formed without movement of the tongue, nor consonants without the tip of the tongue. For as far as it is moveable the tongue divides the voice into distinct words, and as it strikes against either the teeth, or the palate, or the lips, it is believed by the learned to discriminate words accordingly, and to modulate with fineness the sound of speech.

"And for the same reason it is not wonderful that when the tongue, the genuine instrument of articulate voice, had received injury, the voice itself should have been injured likewise; but that the same voice, after being mute for three years, should nevertheless have come back to him in a perfect state, while the tongue remained mutilated just as before, is indeed a thing which exceeds the comprehension of all the learned. For he not only was able to utter sounds easily (a power which has been possessed perfectly by others after their tongue has been cut out), but he could clearly distribute his voice into distinct words, and he spoke all of them very articulately."

The whole of Dr. Tulp's remarks on this case are published in the Appendix,[d] in the original Latin. His mode of conceiving what happened to Joannes seems to be that in consequence of what he suffered from the pirates, his tongue was tied, and that the sudden shock from the flash of lightning burst the ligature. But the explanation of what occurred is altogether a separate point from the fact that Joannes was ultimately able to speak. On the present occasion, Dr. Tulp's testimony is simply adduced to show that he once conversed with a man who spoke very clearly, although a considerable portion of his tongue had been cut out.

---

[d] See Appendix E.

3.—*Case of the Portuguese Girl.*

Another instance of a person's speaking without a tongue is attested both by Dr. Joseph Wilcocks—b. 1673, d. 1756—and M. Antoine de Jussieu—b. 1686, d. 1758. Dr. Wilcocks was elected Demy of Magdalen College, Oxford, in 1689, at what was called the Golden Election, with Boulter, afterwards Archbishop of Armagh, and with Addison. He was subsequently chaplain to the British Embassy at Lisbon, then preceptor to the daughters of George II., then Bishop of Gloucester, and, finally, during the last twenty-five years of his life, Bishop of Rochester and Dean of Westminster. M. Antoine de Jussieu was the first distinguished member of a well-known French family, whose name is now inseparably connected with the science of botany. He was a physician in considerable practice, Director of the Botanical Garden at Paris, and at an early age Member of the Institute. The case, which they both attest independently, is that of a Portuguese young woman, native of Monsaray in the province of Alemtejo, a fortified town on the Guadiana, eight leagues east of Evora. She appears to have been born without a tongue. Her name is not mentioned, but both Dr. Wilcocks and M. Antoine de Jussieu conversed with her, and each has left on record the result of their observations; the former in a letter written from Lisbon while he was Chaplain to the Embassy; the latter in a paper read before the Royal Academy of Sciences at Paris, which has been printed in their Transactions. Dr. Wilcocks's letter is preserved in Wanley's 'Wonders of the Little World,' vol. i. p. 31, edition of 1806. The letter is printed with the date of Lisbon, September 3, 1707 (probably in the original, 1717), and runs as follows:—

"The Conde d'Eiceyra (Conde da Ericeira), a nobleman of letters and curious in natural knowledge, brought from the frontiers of this country a young woman without a tongue who yet speaks very well. She is seventeen years old, but in stature exceeds not one of seven or eight. I was with her at the Conde's house, and made her pronounce every letter of the alphabet, which she can do distinctly, except Q which she calls *Cu*, after the common pronunciation of all her country people. She hath not the least bit of a tongue, nor anything like it; but the teeth on both sides of her under jaw turn very much inward, and almost meet. She finds the greatest want of a tongue in eating; for as others when they eat move their meat with their tongue, she is forced to use her finger. She pretends to distinguish tastes very well; but, I believe, doth it imperfectly. Her voice, though very distinct, is a little hollow, and like that of old people who have lost their teeth. The Conde who is a friend to the Muses, hath written the following epigram on the occasion :—

"Non mirum elinguis mulier quod verba loquatur,
  Mirum est cum linguâ quod taceat mulier."

The memorandum, or report, of M. Jussieu is of still greater importance, as having been presented by a professionally scientific man to a scientific body. I proceed to publish in English some portions of it; but the whole of it may be read in the Appendix,[e] in the original French just as it is printed in the Transactions of the French Royal Academy of Sciences for the year 1718.

"OBSERVATIONS ON THE WAY IN WHICH A GIRL WITHOUT A TONGUE DISCHARGES THE FUNCTIONS WHICH DEPEND ON THAT ORGAN.—By M. DE JUSSIEU.

"I announced, in the month of April last, to Monsieur the Abbé Bignon and to the Academy, in a letter which I had the honour to write to them from

---

[e] See Appendix F. The Conde da Ericeira referred to by Bishop Wilcocks and M. Jussieu was the fourth Count Dom Francisco Xavier de *Menezes*, b. 1673, d. 1743. He was a man of letters, and translated Boileau's 'Art of Poetry' into Portuguese. There is some account of his life in the 'Biographie Universelle,' under *Ericeira;* but none in the valuable 'Nouvelle Biographie Générale.'

Lisbon, the observations which I had made of the way in which a girl born without a tongue discharged all the functions which are performed by that organ. And as my want of leisure did not then permit me to give a full relation of all the circumstances of that phenomenon, I perform my promise now.

"The girl in question was born of poor parents in a village of Alemtejo, a small province of Portugal. She was presented at about nine years of age to the Count of Ericeira (a nobleman as much distinguished by his rank as by his love for letters), when during the last war he entered that province as a commander of part of the troops of her Portuguese majesty.

"The novelty of the fact having excited his curiosity, in order to satisfy it at leisure, he sent the girl to his own house at Lisbon, where I saw her twice consecutively, and examined her with all the attention in my power.

"She was then about fifteen years old, and had sufficient intelligence to answer all the questions which I put to her respecting her condition, and on the manner in which she supplied the want of her tongue.

"In the evening by candlelight, and the next morning in broad daylight, I made her open her mouth, within which, in the space ordinarily occupied by the tongue, I merely remarked a small projection of a pap-like form, which rose about three or four lines high from the middle of the mouth. This projection would have been almost imperceptible to me, if I had not assured myself by touching it, of what could scarcely be recognised by the sight. I felt by the pressure of my finger a kind of contraction and dilation, which made me understand that although the organ of the tongue seemed to be wanting, the muscles nevertheless which form it, and are destined for its motions, were there, as I did not see any vacant space under the chin, and I could only attribute to those muscles the alternating movement of that projection.

" Having ascertained the condition of all parts of the mouth in relation to the absence of the tongue, I made a particular examination of the manner in which the girl performed the five ordinary functions for which the tongue is designed.

" The first, which is *speaking*, is performed by her so distinctly and so easily, that one could not believe that the organ of speech is wanting to her, if one were not told of it beforehand; for she pronounced in my hearing not only all the letters of the alphabet, and several syllables separately, but even a series of words forming complete sentences. I remarked, nevertheless, that among the consonants there are some in particular which she pronounces with greater difficulty than others, such as C, F, G, L, N, R, S, T, X, and Z; and when she is obliged to pronounce them slowly or separately, the trouble which she takes to sound them is manifested by a stoop of the head, in which she draws in her chin towards the throat or larynx, as if to raise the latter, and pressing it, to make it come near the teeth, and to bring it to their level.

"The second function of the tongue, that of *tasting*, is exercised by her with nearly the same discrimination of the quality of savours as would be possible for ourselves, as she told me herself that she found an agreeable sweetness in the dried sweetmeats which persons used to give to her.

"It appeared to me that *mastication* was the thing most difficult for her to perform, for that small projection which I have remarked her as having in the lower part of her mouth not being of sufficient extent to bring her solid food between her two jaws, and to push it back there as often as is necessary in order that it may be reduced to pulp, she employs for this function the movement of the lower jaw, which she brings near to or removes from the molar teeth or grinders of the upper jaw, under which is the bit or food which she wishes to chew. She even sometimes makes use of one of her fingers for this purpose.

"But there is no function for which her fingers are of such effectual use to her as for the *deglutition* of solids, in which operation the tongue is so necessary in order to push them into the pharynx, when they have been prepared by mastication, and when the tongue, as a kind of spoon, has collected every bit of food from all sides of the mouth. She principally makes this use of her fingers, either when the portions of food presented to her are more difficult to be chewed, and therefore require more time for the purpose; or when, those portions requiring more saliva in order to be diluted, the salivary glands of the mouth are exhausted, and cannot furnish sufficient liquid to make the food slide easily and of itself into the œsophagus.

"With respect to *drinks*, she only differs in the mode of swallowing them, by the precaution which she takes not to give herself so much as other persons at a time, and to bend her head forward a little, that she may lessen the fall which the liquids would have if she held her head upright, and may thus run less danger of choking herself. Even the projection which is in the middle of her mouth in the place of her tongue is not without its use, to protect the larynx from too great an influx of drink by its acting as a slight obstacle, which compels the drink to divide itself, and to take the ordinary road of liquids.

"With regard to the act of *spitting*, which one cannot speak of as depending absolutely on the tongue, but in which nevertheless the tongue is of so much use that without its use spitting cannot ordinarily be effected—whether by its collecting the serous matter which is separated from the glands of the mouth, or by its disposing in such a way of the saliva which it has collected, and the phlegm which has been rejected by the lungs, that they may easily be rejected far from the mouth by a violent expectoration—with regard, I say to this act, it is true that the small projection is altogether incapable of collecting the saliva in the mouth, and still less of carrying it to the lips. But, to supply this defect, as the lower part of the mouth, filled by the motor-muscles of the small projection, raises itself nearly to a level with the teeth of the lower jaw, and as the cheek muscles come close to the two jaws, these two sets of muscles together press out the serous matter, and conduct it to the sphincter of the lips, whence the air which the girl ejects forcibly from the larynx acts as a vehicle to expel this saliva, which in proportion as it is thicker can be spit out to a greater distance.

"I do not relate this as a new fact, inasmuch as nearly eighty years ago a surgeon at Saumur, of the name of Roland, made similar observations recorded in a small treatise, entitled 'Aglossostomographie,' or description of a mouth without a tongue, which spoke and performed all the other functions depending on that organ, like the mouth of the Portuguese girl. The sole difference between the two cases is that the case recorded by the surgeon is that of a boy between eight and nine years old, who had lost his tongue through a gangrene caused by ulcers which had come upon him in the small-pox, whereas the girl of whom I am now writing came into the world without any tongue at all."

Subsequently, M. Jussieu proceeds to say:—

"If in the five ordinary functions of the tongue which the girl, as I have observed, was able to perform without that organ, there is any one function more worthy of our observations than the rest, it is undoubtedly that of *speaking*, especially since we are assured by the intelligent researches of M. Dodart that the glottis is the organ of the voice, and that sounds modified in divers ways in the mouth form speech.

"This singular fact of a mouth which speaks without a tongue ought to serve to persuade us that we cannot conclude that the tongue is an organ essential to speech, since there are other organs in the mouth which concur in this employment of it, and others which supply the place of the tongue.

"The uvula, the ducts of the nose, the palate, the teeth, and the lips, have so much to do with speech that whole nations are distinguished in their manner of speaking by the dominant use of some of those parts.

"With regard to the parts which can supply the absence of the tongue, I have not remarked any more capable of fulfilling this function than the muscles which would have made the tongue act if it had been in the mouth entire. Of these the principal are the genioglossi, which take their rise from the inside of the chin, and go on to insert themselves nearly at the base of the tongue. These are the muscles which, conjointly with the geniohyoids and the mylohyoids, drawing to them the hyoid bone in the direction of the chin, appear to raise the larynx and bring it close to the teeth, so that the space between the two parts being diminished by this contraction, the voice in issuing from the larynx is much less broken than it would be if the cavity of the mouth was greater."

There then follow many intervening observations, and M. Jussieu concludes thus :—

" In conclusion, if I have mentioned in this statement some circumstances which seem to render it conformable to that of the surgeon of Saumur, very far from suppressing them, I have thought on the contrary that after having accurately observed them myself on the subject of this report I ought not to omit any one of them ; so that the possibility of a fact which appeared extraordinary might appear the more strongly verified, and that more and more assurance might be gained, that the parts enclosed in the mouth are so necessary to the act of speech that they can in this function supply the absence of the tongue."

Such is the report of M. Jussieu on the case of the Portuguese girl, which even without the confirmation of his statements by Bishop Wilcocks, seems eminently worthy of credit. Apart, however, from its intrinsic merits, it deserves special notice from its having been referred to in controversy by Dr. Conyers Middleton as far back as 1748. If M. Jussieu's report had then been generally read, and Dr. Middleton's remarks on that report had been fully appreciated, the case of the African confessors would, perhaps, never again have been referred to as miraculous. When I published a memorandum on that case in 1858, I was not acquainted with either Dr. Middleton's remarks or the report of M. Jussieu; but now, as it is evident that Dr. Middleton was the first controversialist who correctly explained the power of speech in the confessors, it is due to him to state fully what he wrote on the subject.

He noticed the case under the following circumstances. Dr. Berriman, a clergyman of the Church of England (b. 1688—d. 1750), had published in 1725 a work entitled, 'An Historical Account of the Trinitarian Controversy.' In that work he adverted argumentatively to the case of the confessors in the following passage, which shows that he entertained an unhesitating conviction on three points; 1st, that their power of speech was a fact; 2ndly, that it was a miracle; and, 3rdly, that he himself knew the precise motives which influenced the Divine Mind in causing the miracle to take place.

" The stupidity of these barbarians made them little

capable of conviction from any arguments that might be drawn either from scripture or antiquity. And, therefore, God was pleased to work divers miracles as well for the conviction of such as were not hardened beyond all remedy, as for the greater support of his faithful servants under that severe trial to which they were exposed. Among the rest there is none more considerable than that of the clergy and inhabitants of Tipasa in Mauritania, who when they could not be prevailed with to profess Arianism and be re-baptized (as was the common practice of the Arians at that time), but continued to celebrate the praises of Christ as consubstantial with the Father, had their tongues cut to the roots by the command of Huneric, and then, by a surprising instance of God's good providence, they were enabled to speak articulately and distinctly without their tongues, and so continuing to make open profession of the same doctrine, they became not only the preachers but living witnesses of its truth.

"I am not insensible that miracles have often been pretended in these latter ages, which may be justly called in question, as being both obscurely performed and insufficiently attested. But this is related with such public circumstances, and attested by such competent witnesses that I see not how we can discredit it without shaking the whole faith of history, and rejecting all accounts of miracles besides the scriptural. It was not the case of any single person, but a great number of the inhabitants of a city well known in Mauritania. It was not the wonder of a day or two; but this faculty of speech continued to the end of their lives, excepting only two persons of their whole number, who for the immorality of their practices were punished by Divine Providence with the loss of that extraordinary favour, which had been bestowed on them for the orthodoxy of their faith. It was not an obscure matter uncertainly reported from a corner of Africk, but many of these confessors travelled to Constantinople itself, where their case was examined by such as knew the world, and whose testimony leaves no ground for suspecting an imposture.

"Procopius of Cæsarea who lived in their time, and was himself a senator of Constantinople, speaks of it as a matter that was public and well known in that place, and has left us his account of the fact under his own hand. So likewise has Æneas of Gaza, who relates in his Dialogue under the person of Axitheus, with what curiosity he had examined into the truth of this strange fact, and opened their very mouths to make his observations with the more exactness. They were seen there by Justinian, who was afterwards emperor, and gave account how he had heard from themselves a relation of their own sufferings. And Marcellinus Comes, who was Justinian's chancellor, has left it likewise under his hand, that he saw 'em there himself, and has added this considerable circumstance, that one of the confessors treated in this manner had all his life been dumb, until the execution of this barbarity. Besides all which we have Victor Vitensis, an African bishop and confessor of those times, not only relating it as a certain fact but referring any one that doubted of it to Constantinople, where one of them was still living, and held in great reverence by the whole court, and particularly by the empress herself. And so again Victor Tununensis, another African bishop who lived after them (as being both bishop and confessor in the reign of Justinian), alleges the testimony of the *royal city* (i. e., Constantinople), where their bodies were interred. Not to insist now on the authority of Gregory the Great, who had his account likewise from an ancient bishop who had actually seen them, and Isidore, archbishop of Sevile, who was contemporary of Gregory and a person of too much learning and judgment to be deceived in so important a fact, which was not a century before him."

It will be observed that Dr. Berriman not only quotes the writers afterwards quoted by Dr. Newman, but likewise appeals to the authority of Isidore, archbishop of Seville. Isidore (b. 570—d. 636), however, who was younger than Pope Gregory I., does not really add much to the weight of testimony in this matter. He wrote in Latin a Chronicon, or chronicle of events from the beginning of the world down to the year 636, and in this he narrates briefly the persecution of the Catholics by Huneric. But what he states of the confessors is merely copied, almost word for word, from the Chronicle of Victor Tunonensis; viz., that Huneric "cut out the tongues of confessors, who with their tongues cut out spoke perfectly to the very end." [f]

In reference to the whole passage of Dr. Berriman, Dr. Middleton, after discussing some of the miracles of the fifth century, wrote in his 'Free Inquiry,' as follows :—

"We have dwelt already so long on the miracles of the fifth century that it must be needless to examine the particular merit of that miracle, which Dr. Berriman has so accurately defended. I shall employ, therefore, but a very few words upon it. The story is this; 'Huneric the Vandal, a Christian prince of the Arian heresy in his persecution of the Orthodox party in Africa, ordered the tongues of a certain society of them to be cut out to the roots; but, by a surprising instance of God's good providence, they were able to speak articulately and distinctly without their tongues, and so continuing to make open profession of the same doctrine, they became not only the preachers, but living witnesses of its truth, and a perpetual rebuke to the Arian faction.' [g] This miracle is

---

[f] Isidori Chronicon. See Appendix A.

[g] See Berriman's 'Historic Account of the Trinitar. Controv.,' p. 327, &c., and Dr. Chapman's 'Miscell. Tracts,' p. 174.

attested by several contemporary writers, who affirm that they had seen and heard some of those confessors *speaking distinctly after they had lost their tongues.*"

"Now it may not improbably be supposed on this occasion, that though their tongues were ordered to be cut to the roots, and are said to have been so cut, yet the sentence might not have been so strictly executed as not to leave in some of them such a share of that organ as was sufficient, in a tolerable degree, for the use of speech. It is remarkable also that two of this company are said to have utterly lost the faculty of speaking, who had been deprived perhaps of their entire tongues; for though this be ascribed to the peculiar judgment of God, for the punishment of the immoralities of which they were afterwards guilty, yet that seems to be a forced and improbable solution of the matter. We are told, likewise, that another of these confessors, *who had been dumb from his birth, yet by losing his tongue with the rest, acquired also the use of speech;* which is a circumstance so singular and extraordinary, that it carries with it a suspicion of art and contrivance, to enhance the lustre of the miracle.

"But to come still more close to the point. If we should allow after all, that the tongues of these confessors were cut away to the very roots, what will the learned doctor say if this boasted miracle which he so strenuously defends, should be found at last to be no miracle at all? The tongue, indeed, has generally been considered as absolutely necessary to the use of speech; so that to hear men talk without it might easily pass for a miracle in that credulous age; especially when it gave so illustrious a confirmation to the orthodox faith, and so signal an overthrow to the *Arian heresy*. Yet the opportunities of examining the truth of the case by experiment have been so rare in the world, that there was always room to doubt whether there was anything miraculous in it or not. But we have an instance in the present century indisputably attested, and published about thirty years ago, which clears up all our doubts and entirely decides the question. I mean the case *of a girl born without a tongue, who yet talked as distinctly and easily as if she had enjoyed the full benefit of that organ*, a particular account of which is given *in the Mémoires of the Academy of Sciences* at Paris, drawn up by an eminent physician, who had carefully examined the mouth of the girl and all the several parts of it, in order to discover by what means her speech was performed without the help of a tongue, which he has there explained with great skill and accuracy. In the same account he refers us likewise to another instance, published about eighty years before, by *a surgeon of Saumur*, of a boy, *who, at the age of eight or nine years, lost his tongue by a gangrene or ulcer, occasioned by the small-pox, yet retained the faculty of speaking* in the same manner as the girl.[h]

"Let our doctor then defend this miracle with all the power of his zeal and learning; let him urge the testimonies of *senators, chancellors, bishops, archbishops, and popes;* of persons *who had too much learning and judgment,* he says, to be deceived in so important *a fact, though they lived an hundred years after it;* of *Æneas* also *of Gaza, who opened their very mouths,* as he tells us, *to make his observations with more exactness.* Yet the humble testimony of this single physician, grounded on real experiment, will overthrow at once all his pompous list of dignified authorities, and convince every man of judgment that this pretended miracle, like all the other fictions which have been imposed upon the world under that character, owed its whole credit to our ignorance of the powers of nature."[1]

It only remains to add that Dr. Newman, in his 'Essay on Ecclesiastical Miracles,' has adverted to the above passage, although it had escaped the notice not only of Gibbon himself, but likewise of several learned writers, such as M. Guizot, Dean Milman, and Dr. William Smith, who have published notes on the work of the great historian. Dr. Newman's criticisms

---

[h] 'Mémoires de l'Acad. des Sciences.' Ann. 1718, p. 6.
[1] Dr. Middleton's 'Miscellaneous Works,' Vol. i., pp. 313-316. London. 1755.

on the passage will be found in the Appendix F. Of these the one most to the point is a passing suggestion that "a person *born* without a tongue, as in the instance to which he (Dr. Middleton) alludes, may more easily be supposed to have found a compensation for her defect by a natural provision or guidance, than men who had ever spoken by the ordinary organ, till they came suddenly to lose it." But this suggestion, which did not meet the case of the Saumur Boy, specified by Dr. Middleton, who lost his tongue when he was eight or nine years old, was a pure speculation, unsupported by experience. To render it of any real weight, some one instance should have been adduced of a grown-up person who had lost his tongue in mature life, and who was not able to speak. Perhaps the most singular part of Dr. Newman's criticisms is his asking Dr. Middleton if he means "to say that if a certain number of persons lost their tongues at the command of a tyrant for the sake of their religion, and then spoke as plainly as before—nay, if only one person was so mutilated, and so gifted, it was not a miracle?" To this question Dr. Middleton, if he had been alive, would have had apparently a complete answer. He would have been entitled to reply: "It is strange you should ask me such a question, after reading the 'Free Inquiry.' I have there stated my unhesitating conviction, grounded on experience, that the pretended miracle of the

African confessors owed its whole credit to our ignorance of the powers of nature, and that the tongue is not absolutely essential to the use of speech. How, then, is it reasonable to suppose that my opinion could be altered on this point by the statement of a fact which I knew from the first, that the confessors lost their tongues at the command of a tyrant for the sake of their religion? How could this change into a miracle a power of speech which was otherwise no miracle at all, and which was simply in accordance with the ascertained laws of nature?"

4.—*The case of Margaret Cutting.*

It will be observed that every one of the cases already mentioned occurred out of England. The publication of the first case known to have occurred in England itself was that of Margaret Cutting, investigated in 1742. Margaret Cutting was a young woman of Wickham Market, in Suffolk, in that year about twenty-four years of age, who had lost the whole of her tongue from cancer when she was about four years old. This case deserves special attention from its having attracted the notice of the Royal Society, and from the exhaustive manner in which that renowned scientific body caused it to be investigated. They published an admirable account of it in their 'Philo-

sophical Transactions' for May, June, and July, 1742:
and then, as some of their members still entertained
doubts on the subject, they returned to the case five
years afterwards, in 1747. In that year one of their
members encouraged Margaret Cutting to come up to
London, and brought her to a meeting of the society,
so that all the members present had an opportunity of
examining her mouth, and of hearing her speak. At
the same time Dr. James Parsons, a physician and
member of the society, made a minute examination
of the young woman, and drew up a detailed report
on the subject for his colleagues, which was printed in
the 'Philosophical Transactions' for October, November, and December, 1747.

The 'Philosophical Transactions' of the Royal
Society thus contain two papers on the case of Margaret Cutting. In consideration of their importance,
I now proceed to reprint them both at full length; and
it may be a pleasure to many to come into mental
contact with so much intelligence and thoroughness,
and such an evident pursuit of truth for its own sake,
as these two documents present to the reader. It
should be mentioned, likewise, as adding to their
value, that they are reprinted from the original
edition of the 'Philosophical Transactions,' which is
not often now to be met with even in public libraries,
much less in the libraries of private individuals. The
usual substitute up to the year 1800 is an abridgment

in eighteen volumes quarto, from the commencement in 1665 to 1800 inclusive. This is in itself a very useful work, and it is amply sufficient for ordinary purposes; but in particular cases, when information is required of the most detailed kind, it is unavoidably inferior in value to the original.

The first memoir was read on the 1st of July, 1742, and is reprinted in vol. xlii. of the 'Philosophical Transactions,' No. 464, pp. 143-153. It is entitled "An Account of Margaret Cutting, a young woman now living at Wickham Market in Suffolk, who speaks readily and intelligibly, though she has lost her tongue." The Mr. Henry Baker, who is mentioned in the commencement of the memoir, was a frequent contributor to the Transactions, and he subsequently, in 1744, obtained the Copley Medal for microscopic investigation into the crystallization of saline particles. He died in 1774, at the age of seventy-eight. The whole of the memoir is now subjoined.

"A brief account of this young woman's case, in a letter from Mr. Benjamin Boddington, of Ipswich, turkey merchant, to Mr. Henry Baker, F.R.S., was communicated to the Royal Society in the month of February last, and appeared so extraordinary that Mr. Baker was desired to make all possible inquiries into the reality of the fact, and lay before the Society what information he should receive in relation thereto.

"In pursuance of this, he wrote to Mr. Boddington,

and begged the favour of him to make the strictest and most critical inquiry he was able into this affair, not only by viewing the young woman's mouth, and examining her himself, but also by calling to his assistance some skilful gentleman in the physical way, and any other learned and judicious person whom he might judge most likely to contribute towards discovering the real truth, and detecting any error, fallacy, or imposition. He likewise desired they would heedfully observe her manner of speaking and articulating the sounds of those letters and syllables, in the formation whereof the apex of the tongue seems more particularly needful. And in order to render their examination more easy as well as satisfactory, he sent a list of letters and sounds, together with several such sentences as he imagined would be most difficult to be pronounced without the help of the tongue.

"Mr. Boddington, as soon after this as their affairs would give them leave, prevailed upon Mr. Notcutt, a minister, a learned and curious gentleman, and Mr. Hammond, who perfectly understands anatomy, to accompany him to Wickham Market, about twelve miles from Ipswich, where the young woman lives; whose case (after they had inspected her mouth, and examined her in the strictest manner), is set forth in the following certificate, signed by them all:—

"'Ipswich, April 9, 1742.

"'We have been this day at Wickham Market, to satisfy our curiosity concerning Margaret Cutting, a young woman who, we were informed, could talk and discourse without a tongue.

"'She informed us that she was now more than twenty years of age, born at Turnstal, a village within four miles of Wickham Market, in Suffolk, where she lost her tongue by a cancer [being then about four years old]. It first appeared like a small black speck on the upper superficies of the tongue, and soon ate its way quite to the root of it. She was under the care of Mr. Scotchmore, a surgeon of Saxmundham, who soon pronounced the case incurable; however, he continued using the best means he could for her relief. One day, when he was syringing of it, the tongue dropped out, and they received it into a plate, the girl, to their amazement, saying to her mother, "Don't be frighted, Mamma, 'twill grow again." It was near a quarter of a year after, before it was quite cured.

"'We proceeded to examine her mouth with the greatest exactness we could, but found not the least appearance of any remaining part of a tongue, nor was there any uvula. We observed a fleshy excrescence on the under left jaw, extending itself almost to the place where the uvula should be, about a finger broad. This excrescence, she said, did not begin to grow till some years after the cure. It is by no means movable, but quite fixed to the parts adjacent. The passage down the throat at the place where the uvula should be, or a little to the right of it, is a circular open hole, large enough to admit a small nutmeg.

"'Notwithstanding the want of so necessary an organ as the tongue was generally supposed to be, to form a great part of our speech, and likewise to be assisting in deglutition, to our great admiration she performed the office of deglutition, both in swallowing solids and fluids as well as we could, and in the same manner; and as to speech, she discoursed as fluently and well as other persons do, though we observed a small sound, like what is usually called speaking through the nose, but she said she had then a great cold, and she believed that occasioned it. She pronounced letters and syllables very articulately: the vowels she pronounced perfectly, as also those consonants, syllables, and words that seemed necessary (sic) to require the help of the tongue, as *d, l, t, n, r, at, al, ath, ash, cha, la, ta, ja*. *The little dog did not eat bread—touch the tooth—try to light the candle—thrice thirty-three—let the large cat scratch the little dog—The church—doth—Lilly*. All these she pronounced perfectly. She read to us in a book very distinctly and plain, only we observed that sometimes she pronounced words ending in *ath* as *et—end* as *emb—ad* as *eib;* but it required a nice and strict attention to observe even this difference of sound. She sings very prettily, and pronounced her words in singing as is common. What is still very wonderful, notwithstanding the loss of this useful organ, the tongue, which is generally allowed by anatomists and natural philosophers to be the chief, if not the sole, organ of taste, she distinguishes all tastes very nicely, and can tell the least perceivable difference in either smell or taste.

"'We, the underwritten, do attest the above to be a true account,

   "'BENJAMIN BODDINGTON,
   "'WILLIAM NOTCUTT, *Minister,*
   "'WILLIAM HAMMOND, *Apothecary.*'

"Mr. Baker received, along with the foregoing certificate, by letter from Mr. Boddington, some further particulars which he supposed less material. He says: In her person she is a little thin body, genteel enough, a pretty good face, fair complexion with light-brown hair, of a weakly constitution, lame on one side, through weakness after a fever and the small-pox which she had last summer. She seems a well-behaved girl, and has nothing of a country mien. She discourses agreeably, very fluently and pertinently, has everything clean and neat about her, gets her livelihood by making mantuas, and has an aunt in London, named Mary Cutting, who is housekeeper to the Dowager Lady Rochfort, in Bond-street.

"He says, if she were among twenty people in a room, he thinks it would be impossible for a stranger by any means to guess her being the person without a tongue, for she has no odd motion of her mouth or lips in speaking; she sings with an easy air, and modulates her voice prettily. He asked her if she did not miss her tongue, or find any inconvenience from the want of it? She answered: No, not in the least; nor could she imagine what advantage he had in the use of his. He inquired how she did to guide her food in her mouth to eat. She replied, very easily, she could eat before, on one side or the other, as she pleased, but could not explain the manner how. He was very observing to see her eat, but could discern no difference from others in the moving of her jaws, or other motions of her face, nor in her swallowing food, or in drinking; she did both very neatly, and had exactly the same motion in her throat as we have in its passing down.

"He was apprehensive the excrescence mentioned in the certificate might in some measure supply the use of a tongue; but she assured him it never moved in the least, and that she spoke as well before it began to grow (which was several years after the cure); and Mr. Hammond convinced him by trying with their fingers and a spoon, that it was quite fixed and immovable. He observes further, that she is in no way assisted by a good set of teeth, for she has but few, those bad, and scarce so high as her gums. He asked her in what part of her mouth her most sensible taste lay? She said, it was all over alike; and, smiling, added, she was afraid she was too nice in that, for, if her butter was not curious, she eat dry bread.

"Mr. Boddington, in another letter to Mr. James Theobald, F.R.S., dated the 14th of April, 1742, after giving an account of this young woman in the manner as before, adds, he can recollect nothing more, except her telling him that though she was able to speak from the very first losing of her tongue, she was not so happy as to her deglutition; for she was unable to swallow anything solid for many months after without its being minced very fine, and then thrust into her throat by a finger; but by degrees, she knows not how, she became able to manage without that help, and could eat anything in the same manner as other persons can. He adds that, in his own mind, he thinks the fleshy excrescence is of great service to her, though she cannot make out in what manner; that, for his own part, he had formerly supposed it as impossible to speak without a tongue, as to see without eyes, and therefore expects many who shall hear this account will continue unbelievers, and think he and his friends are all mistaken, that they do not know what they see, and that their ignorance is the only ground of their admiration.

"While Mr. Baker was making his inquiries, he was informed that Mr. John Dennis, tobacconist, in Aldersgate Street, could give him a full and satisfactory account of this affair. He therefore applied to Mr. Dennis, who assured him in a very civil, candid, and intelligent manner, that he was well acquainted with Margaret Cutting, having many years ago been carried by a gentleman to see her, as a prodigy for being able to speak without a tongue. That he had seen her several times since, commonly calling on her when he travels that way, and carrying some friend or other with him; and at all these times he had inspected her mouth, and was sure she had no tongue; and that last summer, in particular, he and another went to see her; that he would declare this under his hand, and should always be ready to attest the truth of it to anybody or in any manner. He likewise gave an account how she lost her tongue, as he had it from her mother, who died some years ago, and it was exactly as above related; and said he had been told the same by an apothecary also, who had her in hand along with Mr. Dr. Scotchmore.

"The testimony of Mr. Dennis, and the person who saw her with him last summer, is as follows:—

"'March 20, 1741.

"'We, the underwritten, saw Margaret Cutting at Wickham Market, in Suffolk, in or about June last; and, examining her mouth, found she had no tongue, and yet she speaks very intelligibly.

"'JOHN DENNIS,
"'GABRIEL DANIELLS.'

"'Myself saw her in about two or three years after her tongue was lost; had a full account of it from her mother; heard her then speak, and have seen and heard her divers times since, and heard her talk better and better.

"'She was under the care of Dr. Scotchmore, at Saxmundham, Suffolk.

"'JOHN DENNIS.'

"Mr. Dennis (upon Mr. Baker's inquiry) wrote to the young woman herself, acquainting her that many people would not believe it possible for her to speak without a tongue, and desiring she would not be ashamed to give an account of herself under her own hand; in answer to which he received the following letter:—

"'To Mr. John Dennis, in Aldersgate Street.

"'SIR,—This being the first opportunity that I had to answer your letter, I assure you that I have no more tongue in my mouth than I had when you saw me last, which is none; but, thanks be to my God, I have had the happiness to speak ever since it came out, which was when I was about four years old. As for my age now, I cannot rightly tell, but I think I am about twenty-four years old. I would have none suspect the truth of it; for I have no tongue, and can speak very well, and this is from my own hand. I was not ashamed to write about myself, but of my bad writing. So no more, but I am,

"'Your humble servant,
"'MARGARET CUTTING.'

"The case of this young woman is indeed extraordinary,[k] but there are several examples of like nature to be met with in medical writers, and those of the greatest authority; one of which, as it has the attestation of a whole university, cannot be improper to mention here. *Monsieur Drelincourt*, a very noted physician, tells us, in his treatise on the small-pox, of a child, eight years of age, who had lost his tongue by that distemper, and was yet able to speak, to the astonishment of the University of Saumur, in France; and that the University (who, doubtless, had first carefully examined into the truth) had attested it, by drawing up a particular account of the fact, that pos-

---

[k] N.B.—All the original papers are in the Repository of the Royal Society.

terity might have no room to doubt concerning the validity of it. The account is to be met with at large, in the third volume of the 'Ephemerides Germanicæ,' under the title of *Aglossostomographia*.

"Tulpius, too, makes mention of a man who had the misfortune to have his tongue cut out by the Turks, and yet, after three years, could speak very distinctly. He says he went himself to Wesop, a town in Holland, to be satisfied of the truth of it, and found it to be as it was reported. Nay, he does not so much as mention any defect in his speech, but assures us that he could pronounce those letters which depend upon the apex of the tongue, even the consonants, very articulately. And this case is even still the more worthy attention, because the patient could not swallow even the least quantity of food, unless he thrust it into the œsophagus by means of his finger.

"If we go back to earlier times, the Emperor *Justin.*, in 'Cod. Tit. de Off. Præf. Præt. Af.,' says, he had seen venerable men, qui abscissis *radicitus* linguis, pœnas miserabiliter *loquebantur*, whose tongues having been cut out by the roots, they miserably *spoke*, or complained of the *punishments* they had suffered. And again, *Nonnullos alios* quibus Honorichius Vandalorum Rex linguas radicitus præciderat, loquelam tamen habuisse integram, that some others whose tongues Honorichius, King of the Vandals, had cut out by the roots, yet perfectly retained their speech."

Next follows the second memoir, which is printed in vol. xliv. part 2 of the 'Philosophical Transactions,' No. 484, pp. 621–626. The title of it is "A Physiological Account of the case of Margaret Cutting, who speaks distinctly, though she has lost the Apex and Body of her Tongue." It is recorded as having been read on the 17th of December, 1747, and allusion is made in it to the presence at the meeting of Margaret Cutting in person. Dr. Parsons, the writer of this memoir (b. 1705, d. 1770), was an eminent physician of his time, who more than once came before the public as an author.

"GENTLEMEN,—As several of the members of this worthy society were somewhat divided in their opinions concerning what was reported of Margaret Cutting, when they were first informed of her by Mr. Baker,[1] it will be necessary (in order to render her case the better understood) to lay before you the following short particulars, which are the result of an examination made a few days since by Dr. Milward and myself; and which, in general, differs not from the opinion which that learned gentleman and I mentioned to this society upon the occasion, which the science of anatomy necessarily suggested to us at that time. But James Theobald, Esq., a worthy member of the Royal Society, having encouraged her to come to

---

[1] See these 'Trans.' No. 464, Art. ii., p. 143, et seq.

London, and having brought her to this meeting of the society, has now given us all an opportunity of coming at the truth of her case, wherefore I shall now, gentlemen, present you with, first, an account of her present condition; and then, some considerations on the natural state and uses of the tongue, which will show you how far she makes the lips and teeth supply the want of her tongue in speaking; and also a direction to every gentleman present to judge of the case before him.

"*Of her present Condition.*

"The apex and body of the tongue (being the only parts that naturally fill the cavity of the mouth) are entirely wanting in this woman, as closely to the region of the *Os Hyoides*, which is the root of the tongue, as can well be conceived; and which is now situated too low in the throat to be perceived, even when she opens her mouth at the widest.

"But let any one lay the tops of the finger and thumb to the sides of her throat, and let her at the same time pronounce the letter *k*, he will feel the remaining root of the tongue rise toward the roof of her mouth, in order to perform it; however, she cannot keep it there any longer than the moment of thrusting it up, for want of the ligament (which was destroyed with the tongue) that is destined, together with the following muscles, to keep the whole tongue forward in its due situation.

"The *Genioglossi* are a pair of muscles which arise from the fore part of the inside of the lower jaw, and are inserted into the body of the tongue by three different directions: the anterior part is carried forward towards the apex; the posterior runs obliquely backwards towards the root, sending a narrow slip on each side to the corner of the *Os Hyoides;* and the middle part ends about the middle of the tongue.

"Now there are certain inequalities appearing on and closely adhering to the floor of the cavity of the mouth, one of which being the most considerable, and having a resemblance in its substance to that of the surface of the tongue, has been, if I am rightly informed, inadvertently mistaken for a tongue by a gentleman professing surgery in the country; and which he thought, for want of a careful examination, performed the offices proper to the apex; but a little care and circumspection would have informed him that those appearances are only fragments of the *Genioglossi* mentioned before, and that upon the separation of the sound parts from those mortified, such fragments as had escaped were retracted and cicatrized down into their present state; nor is it difficult to conceive how the root of the tongue must of necessity sink lower down into the throat, by the loss of these muscles and the proper ligament, which, as I observed before, naturally kept it higher than it could remain ever since their destruction.

"If the mortification had reached the *Os Hyoides*, it must have reached and destroyed the muscles of the *Larynx*, and then the voice would have been destroyed; and also those of the Pharynx, and then deglutition could never have been performed, the dreadful consequences of which need not be enumerated here; but she swallows well, and her voice is perfect, and it is not, therefore, very extraordinary she should command her voice by the proper muscles, which remain untouched.

"The nasal opening is quite exposed, because the uvula which covered it was also destroyed, for one pair of its muscles (the Glosso-Staphilini) arise from the tongue, by which no doubt the distemper was communicated to this part also.

"She has her taste perfectly, which is hereafter accounted for.

"*Some considerations on the natural State and Uses of the Tongue.*

"The tongue is a fleshy substance, chiefly made up of muscles, and consists of a basis or root, a body, and an apex; the basis is the thickest and most substantial part, contains the *Os Hyoides*, and is naturally situated very low in the throat, from which the body rises upwards and forwards, and is terminated by the anterior part or apex, proceeding under the uvula and roof, and lying upon the floor (if I may so call it) of the mouth. As to the more particular description of all its other parts, I cannot apprehend it is at all necessary here, since it is not to our purpose, and would take up too much of your time.

"As to its uses, it is said to be the instrument of *speaking* and *tasting;* as to the latter, experience shows us that the very apex of the tongue is less capable of discerning tastes than the next part to it, and this than the tastes yet farther back, all along the body to the root; so that, although the taste of anything is first perceived by the apex, yet the gust increases the more the morsel approaches to deglutition, until it is quite protruded into the gula, because, as the tongue grows more thick backwards, it contains more of the nervous papillæ than the smaller part, and also because there is a capacity of tasting in the membranes of the back part of the roof to the root, as if nature intended to increase the gust, that deglutition may be the better and more eagerly performed for the service of the animal. Hence, although the apex and body of the tongue be gone, yet there is not a deprivation of taste, which is the case of the person now under your consideration.

"As to *speech*, which is only sound or voice articulated into expression, the tongue is not the sole organ for such articulation; the *lips, teeth,* and *roof* of the mouth are instruments also for the same purpose—the two latter for the necessary resistance to the apex of the tongue, and the lips for the absolute articulation and pronunciation of many letters. However, the following short examination of the letters of the alphabet, as expressed by these organs, will demonstrate it.

"The tongue expresses some letters with its apex and some with its root.

"Those absolutely proper to the apex are only five—*d, l, n, r, t.*

"And those to which it only assists are the following letters, as *c, g, s, x, z,* all which can be performed by the teeth alone, and which this person does very well.

"Now the lip-letters, and those expressed by the root of the tongue, she also performs as well as any person. The former are *b, f, m, p,* and the latter are *k, q, x;* and as to the vowels and the aspiration *h,* since they are chiefly sounded by the exhalation of the voice, commanded partly by the lips in widening or straitening the capacity of the mouth, these she can also express, so that there is no letter she cannot pronounce but the five apex letters, and those she manages so well, by bringing the under lip to her upper teeth, in the course of her conversation, that any one can instantly apprehend every word she says; and she further plainly proves the lips are a better *suc-*

cedaneum to the *apex*, than that could be to the lips if they were wanting.

"Indeed, it is natural enough for those who make the tongue the absolute and sole instrument of speech, to imagine it as absurd to say a woman spoke without a tongue, as that she saw without an eye ; but when we consider the provisional assisting organs ordained by the wise Author of Providence, serving to this necessary and expressive accomplishment, I hope it will not seem so extremely marvellous that she speaks without the body and apex of her tongue, as to create any further doubt of the matter.

"I am, Gentlemen,
"Your most humble Servant,
"JAMES PARSONS."

It will be seen from the concluding paragraphs of the first memoir that reference is made in it to the Saumur case, and the case recorded by Dr. Tulp. Moreover, there is an allusion in it to the African confessors and to the edict of Justinian, in conjunction with those two cases, so that if that memoir had been read attentively and intelligently, in connection with the report of Dr. Parsons, and had been publicly noticed by divines, it ought to have given a death-blow to the idea that there was anything miraculous in the speech of the confessors. It is probable that Dr. Middleton had not read the report of Dr. Parsons until he had published his 'Free Inquiry,' in 1748. At least there is the following statement in a letter written by him, dated the 16th of January, 1749, the year before his death : [m]—

"In drawing up my remarks on that miracle which Berriman defends, I had got a notion of some objections made to the reality of that case of the Ipswich woman, so as to render it of dubious credit, which made me unwilling to venture upon it. But I have since been convinced that the fact was indisputably attested, and that the Transactions of the Royal Society would have supplied an instance as strong and direct to my purpose as that which 1 borrowed from the French Academy."

5.—*Case attested by Sir John Malcolm.*

After the final mention of Margaret Cutting in the 'Philosophical Transactions' of 1747, no one seems to have recorded a case of speech without the whole tongue until the late Sir John Malcolm, in the year 1828, in his 'Sketches of Persia,' mentioned the case of Zâl Khan of Khist. Sir John Malcolm (b. 1769, d. 1833), who was at one time Governor of Bombay, is well known, not only as a distinguished Indian

---

[m] Middleton's 'Miscellaneous Works,' vol. i. p. 419.

administrator, but likewise as an author of various works, and, among them, of a 'History of Persia.' One of the circumstances which led him to undertake the composition of his history was his familiar acquaintance with the Persian language, and the knowledge of Persia and its inhabitants which he derived from having been several times sent to that country by the East India Company on special missions. Indeed, on two occasions, he represented the Company there as their minister plenipotentiary. After he had published his history he published anonymously a small work called 'Sketches of Persia,' which contained some notices of that country and some incidents in his missions which did not come within the range of his history, but which were more or less instructive or amusing. Extracts from his diaries, or note books, evidently form the basis of this work. From various causes he did not put his name to it, but it is known to have been written by him, both from internal evidence and on the authority of his publisher. His mention of Zâl Khan arises in this way. In these 'Sketches' he gives an account of his publicly entering Teheran (apparently in 1800) as minister plenipotentiary, and of his becoming the guest of Hajee Ibrahim, prime minister of Fatteh Ali Shâh, the then reigning sovereign of Persia. In the house of Hajee Ibrahim he became acquainted, and often conversed with, Zâl Khan, chief of Khisht, a village east of Bushire (Abusheher) situated in a small valley near the top of one of the mountains which overlook the arid flat country between their base and the shores of the Persian Gulf. Zâl Khan's tongue had been mutilated by order of Aga Mahomed Khan, the uncle and predecessor of Fatteh Ali Shâh, and Sir John Malcolm mentions the tongue as having been cut close to the root, and, in fact, he speaks of it as not existing at all, and yet he deposes to the fact that Zâl Khan's voice, though indistinct and thick, was intelligible to persons accustomed to converse with him.

The following is the whole passage on this subject referring to Zâl Khan:—

"This remarkable man had established a great name in his native mountains, betwixt Abusheher and Shiraz, and he was long distinguished as one of the bravest and most attached followers of the Zend family. When the death of Lootf Ali Khan terminated its power, he, along with the other governors of provinces in Fars, submitted to Aga Mahomed Khan. That cautious and cruel monarch, dreading the ability, and doubtful of the allegiance of this chief, ordered his eyes to be put out; an appeal for the recal of the sentence being treated with disdain, Zâl Khan loaded the tyrant with curses. 'Cut out his tongue,' was the second order. This mandate was imperfectly executed, and the loss of half this member deprived him of speech. Being afterwards persuaded that its being cut close to the root would enable him to speak so as to be understood, he submitted to the operation, and the effect has been that his voice, though indistinct and thick, is yet intelligible to persons accustomed to converse with him. This I experienced from daily intercourse. He often spoke to me of his sufferings, and of the humanity of the present king (Patteh Ali Shâh), who had restored him to his situation as head of his tribe, and governor of Khisht.

"I am not an anatomist, and cannot therefore give a reason why a man who could not articulate with half a tongue should speak when he had none at all; but the facts are as stated, and I had them from the very best authority, old Zâl Khan himself."

It was the perusal of this passage which first led me to pay special attention to the explanation of the power of speech in the African confessors.

6.—*Case attested by Mr. Wood, British Consul-General at Tunis.*

In 1832 Mr. Richard Wood, now the British Consul-General at Tunis, being then in the public service in the Lebanon, heard the Emir Faris, whose tongue had been mutilated, speak distinctly enough to be understood.

The following were the circumstances under which that mutilation had taken place. The Emir Beshir Shehaab, born in 1764, a man of remarkable ability, by no means cruel in character according to oriental ideas, but fiercely stern towards those who resisted his power, was Prince of the Lebanon, with varying fortunes, from 1788 to 1840. In 1824 three emirs, his relatives, by name Abbas, Faris, and Soliman, were involved in a conspiracy for the overthrow of his authority. That conspiracy failed, and the emirs lay at his mercy, when he presented to them a document for their signature, by which they were to bind themselves never again, during their entire lives, to endeavour in any way to disturb his government, under penalty of having the pupils of their eyes seared with a red-hot iron, and their tongues cut out. They put their seals to the deed, which was carefully preserved; but with infatuated rashness they embarked not long afterwards in a second conspiracy, which failed like the first. They were seized, pinioned, and taken to the palace of the Emir Beshir, who determined to exact the full penalty of the Bond. What followed is thus described by Colonel Churchill, in his 'Mount Lebanon:'—

"The chief of the police soon made his appearance, and shewed them a paper which they all recognised. The seals of Abbas, Faris, and Soliman were indisputably there—there could be no mistake. Nor, indeed, did the unfortunate emirs endeavour to excuse or palliate their folly, and the Emir Abbas particularly, in the midst of his torments, loudly admitted the justice of their fate. Each emir was held down in a squatting position, with his hands tied behind him, and his face turned upwards. The officiating tefeketchy now approached his victim, and standing over him as about to extract a tooth, forced open his mouth, and darting a hook through the top of the tongue, pulled it out, until the root was exposed; one or two passes of a razor sufficed to cut it out. It is a curious fact, however, that the tongues grew again sufficient for the purposes of speech. A red-hot iron was then passed backwards and forwards across the pupil of the eye, till vision was extinct."—Vol. III., p. 384-5.—'Mount Lebanon: a Ten Years' Residence.' London. 1853.

The Emir Faris, whom Mr. Wood heard speak, was one of those three emirs. Mr. Wood's statement on the subject is contained in a letter dated Tunis, 2nd of December, 1872, which he had the goodness to write to me under the following circumstances:—

I had ascertained that Colonel Churchill (b. 1808, d. 1869) could not have himself witnessed the punishment inflicted on the emirs in 1825, as his first visit to the Lebanon was not earlier than in 1840. But it seemed desirable to ascertain likewise, first, whether the emirs, or any of them, were alive in 1840, so that Colonel Churchill might have conversed with one or more of them; and, secondly, whether any of them had been personally known to Mr. Wood himself. I accordingly wrote to him on these points, and inquired at the same time whether he happened to be acquainted with the precise date of the Emir Beshir's death. Mr. Wood was likely to possess information on these points, for, in addition to his previous official experience in Syria, he had been British Consul at Damascus, of well-known efficiency, during a trying period, from 1841 to 1855. His reply was as follows, in a letter dated Tunis, December 3, 1872.

"The Emir Beshir was sent by us, at his desire, to Malta in 1840, or during the Syrian campaign, in which he took part against us, before he was compelled to surrender. After a stay there of about a couple of years, he requested permission to visit Constantinople with his family, which was accorded—and Broussa was fixed as his future place of residence. He died there at an advanced age, but I do not remember the exact period of his demise, nor that of the Emirs Abbas, Faris, and Soliman, whose tongues he caused to be mutilated.

"In 1832 I saw the Emir Faris at the village of Bou Abdo, in the Lebanon. Notwithstanding the mutilation of his tongue, he articulated distinctly enough to be understood, but, as I never heard that his two relatives were able to do so, I attributed the facility with which the Emir Faris articulated more to the imperfect mutilation to which he was subjected than to any other cause.

"I believe the three emirs were dead previous to the arrival of Colonel Churchill in Syria in 1840, but as he resided a great number of years in the Lebanon, spoke Arabic fluently, and one of his daughters married a near relative of the Emir Beshir, he was well versed in the history of the Lebanon, which gives great weight to his statements."

The second paragraph of this letter is the important part of it for my present purpose, as containing the express testimony of Mr. Wood to his having heard the Emir Faris articulate distinctly enough to be understood, notwithstanding the mutilation of his tongue.

It may be added that, although Colonel Churchill is likely to have been correct in attributing the power of speech to all the three emirs, yet his explanation of their speaking by the statement that their tongues *grew* after the mutilation must be rejected as erroneous. The idea of its being possible for human tongues to grow found favour with some anatomists of the seventeenth century; but it is universally discarded by surgeons at the present day, as unsupported by any known fact in the science of comparative anatomy.

Cases attested by Sir John McNeill.   105

From the manner in which the mutilation of the tongues was related by Colonel Churchill, I believed, in 1858, that he was most probably an eye witness of that operation. This certainly was not the case, and the mistake is a good instance of how unsafe it is to infer from the [n] vividness of a narrative that the narrator must have been himself present as an eye witness. Many unobservant persons, although they had been present, might have described the punishment inflicted on the three emirs less vividly than Colonel Churchill, who could only have known what passed through the description of others.

7.—Cases attested by Sir John McNeill.

In 1857, Sir John McNeill, who had been envoy extraordinary and minister plenipotentiary to the Shah of Persia during a period of six years, from 1836 to 1842, made a statement embracing a wider range of facts than is contained in the preceding testimony of Sir John Malcolm and Mr. Wood. He stated that several persons whom he had known in Persia whose tongues had been cut out spoke so intelligibly as to be able to transact important business, and that he had never happened to meet with a person with his

---

[n] See some remarks on this subject in Smith's 'Biblical Dictionary,' under 'Books of Samuel,' vol. iii. p. 1131.

tongue cut out (although he had met with several) who could not speak so as to be quite intelligible to his familiar associates. He likewise explained very clearly in what sense their tongues could be said to have been cut out. He made it evident that the only part really cut out was the portion of the tongue which was loose in the mouth, so that when Sir John Malcolm used the expression of Zâl Khan's tongue having been cut to the root, he must have used the word root to express the attachments which connect the tongue with the under jaw. Sir John McNeill likewise described the process of cutting off the tongue in Persia, which essentially agrees with Colonel Churchill's description of the way in which that punishment was inflicted on the emirs of the Lebanon. And he threw light on Zâl Khan's submitting to a second operation on the tongue, by mentioning that the conviction in Persia was universal that the power of speech was destroyed by cutting off only the tip of the tongue; but that the power was, to a useful extent, restored by cutting out all that was loose in the mouth.

Sir John McNeill's statements were contained in a letter which he was good enough to write to me in answer to inquiries occasioned by my having recently read Sir John Malcolm's account of his conversation with Zâl Khan. The following was the text of Sir John McNeill's letter, which bore date January 8, 1857:—

"In answer to your inquiries about the power of speech retained by persons who have had their tongues cut out, I can state from personal observation that several persons whom I knew in Persia, and who had been subjected to that punishment, spoke so intelligibly as to be able to transact important business. More than one of them, finding that my curiosity and interest were excited shewed me the stump; and one of them stated that he owed the power of speech to the friendship of the executioner, who, instead of merely cutting off the tip as he was ordered, had cut off all that was loose in the mouth, that is, all that could be amputated by a single cut from below. The conviction in Persia is universal that the power of speech is destroyed by merely cutting off the tip of the tongue, and is, to a useful extent, restored by cutting off another portion as far back as a perpendicular section can be made of the portion that is free from attachment at the lower surface.

"Persons so circumstanced appear to me to use the arched portion of the tongue which is behind the point of section as a substitute for the whole tongue, or rather for the tip. This precluded the articulation of certain consonants, but guttural substitutes came to be used, which after a little intercourse, when one had found out the key, as in the case of persons with defective palates, became quite intelligible.

"I never happened to meet with a person who had

suffered this punishment, who could not speak so as to be quite intelligible to his familiar associates. I have met with several of them.

"The mode in which the operation is performed as a punishment will pretty nearly determine how much of the tongue is removed in those cases in which it is said to be cut out by the root. It was described to me as follows, both by persons who had suffered and by others who had witnessed it. A hook was fixed in the tongue near the point, by means of which it was drawn out as far as possible, and then cut off on a line with the front teeth—one man said within the mouth, just behind the front teeth."

On the receipt of the above letter, I forwarded it with a copy of the statements of Sir John Malcolm and Colonel Churchill to the late Sir Benjamin Brodie, with a request that he would favour me with his observations on the subject. Sir Benjamin Brodie (b. 1783—d. 1862), who naturally took more than ordinary interest in a question connected with the profession of which he had been so distinguished an ornament, at once sent to me the following memorandum, dated the 10th of January, 1857.

"There seems to me to be nothing very mysterious in the histories of the excision of the tongue.

"The modification of the voice forming articulate speech is effected especially by the motions of the soft palate, the tongue, and the lips; and partly by the teeth and cheeks. The mutilation of any one of these organs will affect the speech as far as that organ is concerned, but no farther; the effect being, therefore, to render the speech more or less imperfect, but not to destroy it altogether.

"There is no analogy in the higher orders of animals justifying the opinion that the tongue grows again after it has been removed.

"The facts which have been mentioned bearing upon this question are thus easily explained.

"The excision of the whole tongue, the base of which is nearly as low down as the windpipe, is an impossible operation. The eastern executioner, however freely he may excise the tongue, always leaves a much larger portion of it than he takes away. In the healing of the wound, the tongue necessarily contracts from side, it being a rule that the cicatrix of any wound is always smaller than the wound itself. If the tongue be thus contracted in its transverse diameter, it must be elongated in the longitudinal diameter; and hence it would appear when the healing is completed, to project farther forwards than it did immediately after the wound was inflicted."

The most important part in this memorandum is Sir Benjamin Brodie's statement that the excision of the whole tongue is an impossible operation. This must be taken in connection with the context, in which he evidently is referring to the excision of the tongue through the aperture of the mouth, as that operation had been described by Sir John McNeill and Colonel Churchill. With this limitation, his statement commends itself at once to the reason, when the length of the tongue is distinctly apprehended; and it thus becomes evident that the unfortunate persons whose tongues are said to have been cut out by oriental executioners, still retained in their mouth a certain portion of their tongues.

8.—*Cases attested by Dr. Wolff, the Missionary.*

Another witness to the fact of speech without the tongue is the late Dr. Joseph Wolff, the celebrated missionary (b. 1795—d. 1862). As will have been seen from the last case, Sir John McNeill knew many persons without tongues in Persia who spoke so intelligibly as to be able to transact important business; but Dr. Wolff states what at first sight might appear even still more improbable, that in 1824 a priest at Bussorah (or Bassorah), whose tongue had been cut out, actually gave him instruction in a language. This fact is related in Dr. Wolff's 'Travels and Adventures,' a work which was written in the third person under his dictation, and which was first published in two volumes, octavo, in 1860. To render the passage in which it is related fully intelligible, it is proper to mention the following circumstances, which are extracted from Dr. Wolff's work.

There is a sect at Bussorah and elsewhere who call themselves followers of John the Baptist. They regard themselves as descended from Abraham's brothers, and their tradition is that in the course of time their ancestors, who had settled by the River Jordan, received baptism from the prophet whose name they bear. Others give them the nickname of "Sabeans," which means "those who have changed their religion, and turned in their prayers towards the North;" but they call themselves by two names, 1st, Mandaye Haya, *i. e.*, followers of the living God, and, 2nd, Mandaye Yahya, *i. e.*, followers of John (the Baptist). Their language which is Chaldean, with characters entirely their own, is called Mandaye. They have two kinds of priests. One is supposed to represent Jesus Christ and is called Ganz Aura, "he that is acquainted with the whole book," while the other is called "Tameeda," *i. e.*, "the awakened out of sleep," and is supposed to represent John the Baptist. Every Sunday they baptize their followers, and on these occasions the Ganz Aura is baptized by the Tameeda. As will be seen from the following passage the Ganz Aura instructed Dr. Wolff in Mandaye. On Dr. Wolff's authority the word Rabbi, as printed in his Travels, has been changed to Rabba.

"Rabba Adam, the Ganz-Aura priest, was an extraordinary man. He practised magic; and a Muhammadan lady who wished to have a child, came to him, so he wrote some illegible words upon her stomach. The Muhammadan governor heard of this, and got Rabba Adam's tongue cut out, and his right arm cut off; but Rabba Adam cut out the remainder of the tongue which had been left, and then he spoke again.

'Although this sounds quite incredible—so much so that Colonel Taylor advised Wolff never to relate it (although he was a witness to it himself)—it is nevertheless a strict fact. And the same thing happened to a relation of the Prince Beshir in Mount Lebanon, whose tongue was cut out, for by a further excision he recovered the power of speech. Of course these people spoke with difficulty, but they were quite articulate, and Rabba Adam used to come to Wolff daily, and taught him the Sabean, called the Mandaye, language, though without his tongue, and he wrote all he had to write with his left arm. Wolff gave this account to several persons in Malta, who repeated it to Sir Frederick Cavendish Ponsonby, the Governor of Malta, and he said, 'I will believe anything that Wolff says, for he has already told me several things which sounded most incredible, but which turned out to be completely true.'"

In reference to this passage I was afterwards placed

in communication with Dr. Wolff, in March 1861, and I had the pleasure of becoming personally acquainted with him. In answer to questions, he gave me the following additional information respecting Rabba Adam; viz., that he was about fifty-six years of age in 1824, that he submitted to the second operation on his tongue only one day after the first operation, and that, as far as an opinion could be formed by an unscientific observer, he had not the slightest remains of a tongue. Dr. Wolff added that the Rabba could pronounce with some hesitation every Arabic letter except the Ghain, ع.

In the extract from Dr. Wolff's work it will be seen that he speaks of a relation of the Prince Beshir in Mount Lebanon who had the power of speech, though his tongue had been cut out; but it is left somewhat uncertain whether Dr. Wolff himself conversed with him. I specially questioned Dr. Wolff, however, on this point, and he assured me that he spoke from personal knowledge, having been acquainted with the Prince Beshir's relation without knowing his name—that the relation was about twenty-five years of age, and that about three days had intervened between the first and second operation on his tongue. This relative was probably one of the three emirs mentioned in case No. 6; but whether he was or was not the Emir Faris with whom Mr. Wood conversed, is uncertain. In regard to the young man's pronunciation, Dr. Wolff made precisely the same statement as regarding the pronunciation of Rabba Adam, and he believed that both of them were unable to speak a word after the first operation.

In reply to questions whether he had met anyone else in the East whose tongue had been cut out, Dr. Wolff stated that at Bokhara there were above thirty persons who spoke without tongues, and that he had conversed with about twenty of these, either on his first or on his second visit to that city. He said he could give no details of these cases, as he had not directed any special attention to the subject, and his mind was occupied with other matters, when he was at Bokhara.

It may be added that Dr. Wolff was an attractive person with great simplicity and evident veracity of character; and it seemed to me that, although he might accept too readily the statements of others, his own statements might be regarded as thoroughly trustworthy, when he spoke from personal observation of facts respecting which he could not easily be mistaken.

9.—*Cases attested by Mr. Dickson, Physician to the British Legation at Tehran.*

Mr. Joseph Ritchie Dickson, Physician to the British Legation at Tehran, is another witness as to the power of speech remaining in persons commonly said to have been deprived of their tongues. He was in England in the spring of 1859, when I had the opportunity of making his acquaintance, and I was in hopes that on his return to Tehran, he might be enabled to obtain conclusive evidence as to how far the prevalent belief in Persia, as to the effect of merely cutting off the tip of the tongue, was founded on facts which would bear the scrutiny of a European physician. Accordingly, with his most willing concurrence, I sent to him a letter in March 1859, enclosing a statement of various points for minute inquiry in this manner.

Happily for Persia, the punishment of mutilation of the tongue had become rare in that country, and Mr. Dickson did not find himself able to obtain all the desired information. A minute scientific inquiry would in fact have been attended with numerous difficulties, even if mutilation of the tongue had continued to be a common punishment. Still, in August 1862, after full acquaintance with the case of Mr. Rawlings, I wrote again to Mr. Dickson in reference to my previous inquiries. The following year I received from him the following letter with its enclosure. It is dated "Tehran, January the 29th, 1863."

"By the post from Baghdad I had the pleasure of receiving your kind letter dated August the 27th,

1862, which had been a long time on the road, having been sent to Bombay *viâ* Egypt, and back by the Persian Gulf to Baghdad, and from thence to this place.

"I have really to apologise for not having fulfilled ere this my promise of answering, on my arrival here, certain questions respecting the phenomena connected with mutilated tongues, which you transmitted to me in your letter, dated London, March the 28th, 1859.

"The mutilation of the tongue as a punishment is now very rarely practised in Tehran, and the only information I have been able as yet to obtain on this subject, I now beg to transmit to you in the enclosed statements made to me by Mehdee Kooly Beg and Mohammed Sadik.

"The belief in Persia is universal, as Sir John McNeill states, that the power of speech is destroyed by merely cutting off the tip of the tongue, and is to a useful extent restored by cutting off all that is loose in the mouth.

"Mehdee Kooly Beg not only confirms this in his statement, but adds that, convinced of the truth of this belief, and finding that he was speechless after having had the tip of the tongue cut off, he at once performed the operation on himself, and cut off all that was loose in the mouth, and that he was able to speak immediately after.

"According to his statement, both Poolad Khan and Mohammed Rakeem Khan, who had the tip of their tongues cut off, were never able to speak at all distinctly.

"Mohammed Sadik, the young shoemaker examined by me to-day, in his statement says that the whole of the loose portion of his tongue had been cut off, and that he never lost his power of speech. But on examination I found that his tongue appeared very like that of tongue-tied infants, and had a great power of raising or moving forward the base, which gave it the appearance as if it had not suffered any great diminution in bulk. Hence, perhaps, the vulgar notion that the tongue grew again."

The following were the two detailed statements enclosed to me by Mr. Dickson. Each was written down in the third person.

The first was the subjoined statement of Mehdee Kooly Beg :—

"Mehdee Kooly Beg, æt. 50, is of Arabian origin; his tribe was brought from Arabia to Khorassan (in Persia) by Nadir Shah.

"In Fat'h Ali Shah's time, he was 'Naijeb Mirakhor' (Deputy Master of the Horse), under Isah Khan the Mirakhor. At present he is employed at court as Naijeb Ferash Khaneh (Deputy in the Office of Carpet-Spreaders) of the late 'Valiahd,' heir-apparent.

"About thirty-two years ago, at the age of eighteen, having in the king's presence made use of abusive language towards his chief, Fat'h Ali Shah immediately ordered his tongue to be cut off. The executioner claimed fifty tomauns (£25) to perform the operation well, which he refused to give, and therefore only the tip of his tongue was cut off. No sooner was the order carried into effect, than the Shah said that he was pardoned. The poor man, hearing this, made an attempt to ask what was said, but found that he was speechless. He then immediately got hold of a razor belonging to a barber who happened to be present, and cut off the whole loose portion of his tongue. The right side not having been properly cut off, a slight unevenness or protuberance exists which prevents his speaking more distinctly, of which, were it pared off, he says he should be able to speak more clearly. He was able to speak after the second operation.

"He spoke rather thick, but quite intelligibly, with the exception of the following consonants, which he pronounced imperfectly—viz., the letter D he pronounced B; L he could not pronounce; N he pronounced M; R he pronounced like a Parisian; T he pronounced P; and V he could not pronounce.

"Mehdee Kooly Beg also stated that Poolad Khan Bahtyari and Mohammed Rakeem Khan Karachooloo Koord, both had the tip only of their tongues cut off at the 'Nigaristan' palace, by order of Zillah Sultan, son of Fat'h Ali Shah, while Governor of Tehran, when Fat'h Ali Shah went to Sultaniah.

"Both these two Khans were of an advanced age; they did not submit to the operation of cutting off all the loose portion of the tongue, and they were never able to speak at all intelligibly. Only those accustomed to their expressions could understand them."

The second statement was that of Mohammed Sadik. It appears to have been made to Mr. Dickson not more than two years after his tongue had been cut off:—

"Mohammed Sadik, æt. 24, shoemaker, in the year 1861, having been accused of using abusive language in a state of intoxication, was forthwith taken before the Governor of Tehran, Prince Firooz Mirza, Nusret Ed-Dowlah, and condemned to have his tongue cut off. Immediately after the operation he spoke a few words, but soon fainted away, profuse hæmorrhage having taken place. He gradually got well, and now, with the exception of the letter 'r,' he can speak quite distinctly as if nothing had happened to him."

10.—*Case of Mr. Rawlings.*

The next case is that of Mr. Robert Rawlings, an Englishman (b. 1825, d. 1863), who spoke intelligibly although he submitted in 1861 to an operation by which the whole body of his tongue had been removed. He had been first a soldier in the Grenadier Guards, and then an official connected with railways, but he was obliged to give up his employment from ill-health. His disease was cancer of the tongue, and the operation which was had recourse to as affording the only chance of saving his life was performed by the late Mr. Thomas Nunneley (b. 1809, d. 1870), lecturer on surgery in the Leeds School of Medicine, and senior surgeon to the Leeds General Eye and Ear Infirmary. This case differs apparently from all instances of persons whose tongues are cut off in the East; for the operation is described as being performed on them through the aperture of the mouth, whereas in Mr. Rawlings the excision took place under the chin between the lower jaw and the hyoid bone. Early in 1862 my attention was drawn to the case by accidentally reading an account of it in an American newspaper. This led to my instituting some inquiries through Mr. James Garth Marshall, of Headingley Hall, near Leeds; to whose intelligent interest in the subject I am indebted for valuable information communicated by Mr. Nunneley, and likewise for becoming acquainted, through

Mr. Nunneley, with Mr. Rawlings. I conversed with Mr. Rawlings several times, and on my first interview I took down from his lips a short account of his previous life. At my request he submitted himself for examination to some eminent men of science in London, each of whom was willing to make some statement in writing of what he had heard and seen. There is thus so much evidence on record in this case that, though it stood absolutely alone, it would be sufficient to prove that even the removal of the body of the whole tongue is compatible with the faculty of speech. This evidence shall now be set forth in due order.

1. Mr. Nunneley operated on Mr. Rawlings at the end of October and beginning of November, 1861. He naturally kept notes of the case, and as he was a member of the Royal Medical and Chirurgical Society of London, he wrote a long memoir on the subject for that body. It was received on the 14th of November, and read at one of the regular meetings of the society on the 10th of December, 1861; and an abstract of it was published in the first number of the 'Proceedings of the Society,' printed in 1862. Mr. Nunneley furnished me with a copy of the memoir which contains some interesting details not contained in the abstract. As the memoir is the original document, I insert the whole of it, in order to give the amplest possible information respecting this case.

"An Account of a Case in which the entire tongue was successfully removed, for cancer of the organ, by Thomas Nunneley, F.R.C.S., Lecturer on Surgery in the Leeds School of Medicine, and Surgeon to the General Eye and Ear Infirmary.

"The removal of a portion of the anterior part of the tongue, is neither an unfrequent, difficult, nor dangerous operation. It is, however, far different when the whole organ is concerned. Operations for the ablation of the entire tongue have not been frequent, nor are they unattended with difficulty; and the very few cases in which a successful result has followed, fully prove that the operation is of that dangerous character, as only to be justified as an urgent necessity. It is this consideration which induces me to bring before the Society a case in which I have recently successfully performed the operation, under circumstances of considerable difficulty, not only from the extent of the disease itself, but in which the danger was provokingly increased by more than one unforeseen and so to speak extrinsic complication. I would willingly forego a narrative of the details, but I know of no other way in which I can so clearly relate those particulars which are essential to a clear understanding of the case, and my reasons for adopting the course which I did in the progress of it; these however I will curtail as much as possible.

"The difficulty of reaching the extreme base of the tongue so as to excise it by the knife, and the danger of uncontrollable hæmorrhage are so considerable that very few surgeons have been bold enough to attempt it; while those who have experienced and known how great is the difficulty and the amount of force required in applying a ligature so as to effectually strangulate, even a part, if at all considerable, of an organ so freely supplied with nerves and blood-vessels so extensively connected, and in such proximity with important parts as the tongue is, and the long continued agony occasioned by the ligature, will hesitate in adopting the plan when the entire organ is involved.

"It was for the purpose of overcoming these difficulties that Professor Syme was induced, in the only two cases which, so far as I am aware, have recently (if at any time) been undertaken in this country, to divide the lip and soft parts under the chin, and then to split open the lower jaw and retract the sides widely apart before he dissected out the tongue itself (*vide* 'Lancet' for August 1858). Though two operations (as I have learnt since the one now narrated was performed) have been successfully done by a method somewhat similar to that followed by Mr. Syme, by Mr. Fiddes in Jamaica (*vide* 'Edinburgh Medical Journal,' 1859, page 1092, and 'Pathological Transactions' for 1861, vol. xii), the speedy fatal termination from the same cause of both of the cases of Mr. Syme, would, I apprehend, induce most surgeons to pause before repeating the plan, even had Mr. Syme not thought himself called upon to declare that he would not feel himself justified in repeating the operation; for as both of his patients were as favourable subjects as any that would be likely to be presented, and both died from the same cause—diffuse inflammation of the lungs—so in all probability other cases would also terminate. Nor is such a result to be wondered at, when we consider the extensive mischief which the mere operation inflicts upon parts in themselves sound, in addition to the removal of the diseased tongue, in itself sufficiently grave. The splitting of the jaw bone, and the extensive division of such structures, would probably *per se* in a majority of cases be not unattended with danger.

"These considerations are so important that though I think the ecraseur is an instrument which has been often much abused, in being employed in cases for which it is infinitely less fitted than other means, it appeared that if appropriate in any case, provided the chain could be carried far enough back, and fixed securely, the removal of the entire tongue is specially adapted for its employment. I therefore determined to use it—an intention, however, as will be seen by the account of the operation, which the wretched workmanship of the operation prevented being carried into effect.

"R—— R——, æt. 35, is at present a guard, and for several years past has been employed on the Lancashire and Yorkshire Railway; he has been in the police force, and in early life was in the Coldstream and Dragoon Guards. Though now pale and thin, he is a tall, well-built, and formerly was a stout, muscular man. He states that for upwards of two years he has been losing strength, in consequence of being unable to masticate food, owing to disease in the tongue—which commencing three years ago, at first small and confined to one side, has now involved the whole organ. Until this appeared he had uniform good health, and has been certified as a healthy man on three or four occasions when entering societies. When young he was not very steady, but for several years past he has been so. He left the army in 1849, soon after which he married. His wife has had eight children, one being now only six months old; they as well as herself have always been healthy and strong, so that there is no reason to suspect a syphilitic taint. He has been under various medical men for three years past, and subjected to a variety of treatment, including mercurials, and the application of strong caustics, all of which he thinks has done more harm than good: a short time ago two sound molar teeth were extracted, and it was said they stood inwards in consequence of the jaw having been broken many years ago. There is however no evidence of any misplacement in the jaw; all the teeth are natural and in good position; and as the part of the tongue where the disease first made its appearance did not correspond with the alleged faulty teeth, it is more than probable they had nothing to do with its origin.

"When seen by me the whole tongue to its base was found involved, its size was somewhat, though not very greatly, increased, but the entire structure was very hard, dense, and unyielding. In the centre there was a long, deep, narrow ulcer with irregular margins, from which issued an offensive discharge; around this the hardness was very great. From the induration extending unequally towards the edges of the tongue, these were irregular in outline, in some places hard and swollen, in others thinner and more natural. The dorsum was covered with thickened patches. The mouth was filled with saliva, but this appeared to arise rather from the difficulty and disinclination to move the tongue in deglutition than from very decided salivation. There was always a dull uneasy sensation and often sharp lancinating pain. The motions of the tongue were so much impeded that speech was materially interfered with, and so difficult and painful had mastication been for long past, that though hungry he had often been compelled to pass the entire day without taking food, so that he had become very weak. The loss of flesh had been more rapid during the last few weeks. He was so anxious to have something done, that though told the nature of the disease, and the very serious operation he would have to undergo, should operation be decided upon, that he had better take a few days to consider well if he would submit to it; he returned to me in a couple of days saying, as his pain and distress were so great, that he must starve from the difficulty of taking food, he wished the operation to be performed at once.

"Considering the slow progress the disease had made, that though now it had invaded nearly the whole substance of the tongue, yet so far as the position of the parts permitted an examination being made, the extreme base of the organ appeared to be in a natural condition; that death seemed to be the inevitable termination of a life more or less prolonged in great misery, that the difficulty and immediate danger of the operation were not concealed from the patient, who is a man of wonderful nerve, and was willing to undertake the risk, I thought myself justified in giving him what I believe to have been the only chance of recovery.

"*October 1st.*—Having had made an ecraseur, in which by a sliding joint I could detach and securely fasten again one end of the chain to the ratchet-bar, I tied one end of it to a considerably curved needle, of such a size that the chain would easily follow the needle, and then, with the object of being able to carry the chain well back over the base of the tongue, and of having no greater thickness of structure to crush through than could be avoided, having made a transverse incision through the integuments, mylo-hyoid and genio-hyoid muscles just above the hyoid bone, I carried the needle and chain into the mouth, on the left of the median line, close to the side of the base of the tongue, and then brought them out at a corresponding point on the right side of the tongue through the same external aperture under the jaw. The chain was readjusted to the ratchet-bar, and all being ready for the action of the ecraseur, chloroform was given, when just as the instrument was set in motion, before any strain whatever was put upon it, the chain dropped in two, owing to the rivets connecting the links having been filed close away so as to leave hardly any hold; all attempts to secure the broken links and allow the chain to pass through the canula were fruitless, so that the use of the instrument had to be given up.*

"Being fortunately provided with fine well-twisted whip-cord, such as I have used in the partial removal of the tongue, I at once attached a double cord of it to the chain, and withdrawing this carried it into the same place; one of these cords I tied as tightly as I could draw it. To the other I attached a fourfold ligature and drew it across the tongue, feeling sure that one string would be altogether ineffectual. Two of these I used as a double ligature, tightening them with all the force I could exert. The other two I had intended to have kept in reserve for use in a few days, but finding the appearance of the tongue did not indicate complete strangulation, I used them at once with such force, that some of the friends who were assisting me thought I must cut through the substance of the tongue. A stitch was put into the external wound, a grain of acetate of morphia given, and the patient put to bed.

"He suffered greatly at first. As he could neither talk nor swallow I had a strong solution of acetate of morphia made (gr. x. ad ʒ iss of water), so that a few drops might be placed in the mouth from time to time. Injections of beef tea and gruel containing morphia, according to circumstances, were administered. These procured sleep and comparative ease. All went on well for three days, the pain becoming much less and the pulse improving; the worst symptom which supervened after the first forty hours

---

* The instrument was a new one made expressly for me; there was no visible defect in it, and as I had tried it upon a piece of horseflesh larger than the human tongue, I thought I had taken sufficient precaution to test it. I am told that this class of instruments are rarely made by the persons who supply them, but are procured by them from those who technically are said "to work for the trade," but who nevertheless stamp the name of the seller upon the instrument supplied to them.

was a frequent cough and hurried breathing, with tenacious bloody sputa, which, as he could not expectorate, caused some trouble, and excited the suspicion that my patient might suffer from the same form of pneumonia which carried off both Mr. Symes'.

"On the 4th he was so much improved that in the afternoon I not only lessened the strength of the solution of morphia, but directed that he should not have any more until ordered, as I found the dose he had had to be sufficient to relieve the pain. These directions were disobeyed. During the night I was called up with the statement that he was dying, which I found to all appearance too true—poisoned by morphia, two more doses of which had been improperly given to him. He was insensible; the pupils were contracted to a point, the breathing at first stentorious became imperceptible, the pulse was nearly gone, and the extremities and depending parts of the body were livid. As he could swallow nothing by the mouth, and he was in too weak a state to be violently roused, four ounces of a very strong decoction of coffee was given as an enema every quarter-of-an-hour. Contrary to all expectation, after lying in this lethargic condition eight hours, he gradually improved, and by the evening all danger of dying from the narcotic had passed away. The intensity of the narcotism was so great that I was led to an investigation of the composition of the solution, when I found that the too frequent administration of the dose was not the worst error that had been committed, for instead of reducing the quantity of morphia in the bottle from ten to six grains as prescribed, it had been increased to twenty grains, so that within six hours the patient had taken by mouth and anus about four grains of acetate of morphia."

---

[p] The compounder says the mistake arose from a drunken man forcibly intruding himself while the medicine was being

"10th.—Since the last report he has gone on favourably. The cough and threatening of pneumonia have disappeared. His general condition has improved. He has retained the nutritive enemata well, and to-day has swallowed a little broth. The pulse is natural and good. The morphia required is much less than it was, but the tongue, which at first was dark and swollen, has gradually recovered its red hue, is less swollen and much more sensitive. There is a free suppuration from the submental aperture, which, though offensive, has not a gangrenous odour. Though the ligatures have cut so far into the base of the tongue that they can neither be seen nor felt, it is obvious that the strangulation is not sufficient, either from the slackening of the cords, the lessened size of the parts they embrace, or the broad sublingual connection which is unimpeded. I therefore determined to day, if possible, not only to carry another and stronger ligature from under the chin across the base, but also to place one from the deep fissure cut in this under the frænum, so as completely to isolate the organ; and having got some silk whipcord of a blue colour, so strong that a powerful man had tried in vain to break it, I carried, by means of a long probe, a double thread of this, and also a double one of the white flax cord, through the submental

---

prepared, which so irritated him, that he forgot what he was about. How far did leaving the patient quiet conduce to his recovery? It has sometimes struck me that after opium poisoning it is a question if the effects would not sooner pass off, if the patient were less perseveringly roused. If sleep has not already supervened it may be right to prevent it if possible coming on; but I much doubt, if the patient already be in a deep sleep, if it is not better to let him be quiet. I certainly never saw any one so completely narcotized recover, and the rapidity with which all the symptoms passed off after he began to rouse up was unusual.

opening into the mouth on each side of the tongue along the course of the former threads. This I was obliged to do, as it was impossible to carry a cord across the tongue from without to within, and then from within to without, as the parts were too tender and swollen to admit of it. By having one cord blue and the other white, the securing of the corresponding ends to each other was much facilitated. I then divided the cords so as to have each end separate, and having drawn one of each kind, one on each side, well out of the way so as to have them in reserve for a future time, I tied the other four ends together in a firm knot, and carried this into the fissure already made in the base of the tongue. Chloroform was now given, and then the outer cords of the stronger silk cords, already twisted round pieces of wood so as to obtain a better leverage than the hands alone could afford, were drawn so tightly that just as the knot was made one of them broke, but fortunately so as not to interfere with its holding. The thinner cord was now very carefully placed along the whole breadth of the fissure, and brought round the margin of the tongue underneath the frænum, where it was tied as tightly as possible, the connection of it with that carried from the fissure under the chin effectually prevented its slipping forwards, as it otherwise would have been liable to have done, and thus cutting obliquely and partially, and not through the whole substance of the tongue, which now was completely encircled. In tying the cords, it was evident that the structures were much softer, as they were felt to yield much more than they did before, and some bloody pus of a gangrenous odour was forced out. The tightening of the cord under the frænum produced a much more marked effect upon the appearance of the tongue than did that under the chin. Though the pain was severe at the time, it was controlled by much smaller doses of morphia, and was much sooner mitigated than after the first operation.

"*14th.*—He has considerably improved in all respects; he sleeps well, has no very urgent pain, and can swallow sufficient liquid food and wine. Yet though there is a decided gangrenous odour, the tongue is becoming again more natural in size and appearance.

"*15th.*—Soon after midnight there was copious bleeding from the mouth; when I got to him he had lost nearly a pint of moderately dark blood. It was impossible to see the exact spot from whence it came. The mouth was repeatedly filled with a mixture of one part of the tincture of the sesquichloride of iron and two of water, with the effect of speedily arresting the hæmorrhage; after which he slept well, and had no return of the bleeding till this afternoon, when it was at once stayed by the solution of muriate of iron. In the evening the hæmorrhage returned more copiously, when, fearing the effect of the muriate of iron upon the ligatures, I used a strong solution of tannic acid, which was not only put into the mouth but was also injected along the course of the threads from the submental opening, the bleeding was immediately arrested. Though not many ounces of blood were lost on this occasion or during the afternoon, he was considerably reduced by it.

"*16th.*—No more bleeding; he has taken food well, and rallied considerably.

"*17th.*—The bleeding again recurred during the night, but was at once checked by the tannin. As afterwards there was a renewed tendency to it, I tied the reserve ligature round the base of the tongue, which, though it had been weakened so as to give way before nearly so great a strain was put upon as on the last occasion, the effect upon the appearance of the tongue was marked, and the bleeding was stopped.

"*19th.*—Since the last ligature was tied he has most materially rallied in strength, and there has not been any more of the bleeding until this evening (fifty-four hours), when it returned so freely that I again placed ligatures, in the same manner as on the 10th instant, through the submental opening over the base of the tongue, and also under the frænum. As I feared either the knots had not been drawn home, had given way, or that the cord was too thick to compress closely, I employed another material, and one which, so far as I know, has not before been made use of as a ligature, but which, where strength, sharpness, and fineness are of importance, promises to be of great value, since it possesses these properties in a greater degree than any other substance I am acquainted with. I had obtained it before the silk ligatures were used on the 18th, but as on submitting it to a microscopic examination I found it to be an animal tissue, I feared that it might soon soften in the fluids, and so give way. Having, however, then placed some of it in water, and kept it until the present time in a warm room, without any change in it being perceptible, I ventured to employ it. Judging from the yielding of the tissues, and the appearance of strangulation, I should imagine it has acted well, and that not much remains to be cut through.[a]

"23rd.—He has gone on favourably in every respect,

---

[a] I cannot learn the name or nature of this cord. I got it from a fishing-tackle dealer, who tells me he believes it comes from China, and would be invaluable as a fishing line did it not curl so much in the water—a quality which is the only drawback against its employment as a cutting ligature—as this renders its application in deep cavities somewhat difficult. Though it is certainly an animal tissue, its non-imbibition of water is remarkable. I exhibit a portion which has been kept for a month immersed in water in my library. Its twist is something altered, and its strong tendency to curl is lessened, but neither its strength nor size is altered in any material degree.

except the non-separation of the tongue, till last night, when an ounce of blood was lost; during the night the hæmorrhage recurred three times, and again this morning. Though on each occasion it was at once arrested by the solution of tannin, he was so greatly exhausted that I again placed ligatures round the base under the frænum, using the same material as last time. Though reserve ligatures were in place, fearing they might be weakened by the teeth or decomposition, I introduced fresh threads. The tongue at once again assumed a leaden hue, which it had been losing. So little pain was occasioned this time, that it is evident the lingual nerves must have been already cut through.

"30*th*.—Since the last report he has not had an unfavourable symptom, nor return of the bleeding. He can sit up for an hour. There has been so little pain that he can sleep without the morphia, and says if the tongue were only away so that he could masticate, he could enjoy a beefsteak. Though the hue of the tongue has become more natural, it has lost all sensation. There is a free escape of fœtid pus. Though pulled and twisted daily, the ligatures are still firm, I have therefore placed others in the two places—the tongue becoming quite livid. Not the least pain was caused, and as the mouth could be better opened, the ligatures could be carried across the tongue without the intervention of a knot.

"*November 2nd.*— Since the application of the last ligatures, the tongue has become much more swollen, particularly on the right side; and as the base of the tongue appeared to be completely cut through, although the ligatures were still fast on the sublingual tissues, in the hope of separating it altogether, I have to day carried from the fissure under the frænum a well-twisted double suture (Simpson's) wire, by means of a rod having a short and long transverse arm, with holes in, through which the wire was passed, so that it could be tightly twisted close to the tongue. This was done until the wires gave way, without severing the tongue. On the 3rd, I repeated the wire ligature, but this time a strong pianoforte string was used. The tongue became quite dark and loose, and was forced between the teeth, but just as I thought it would be separated, the wire gave way, leaving some connection still remaining.

"On the 4th, as no pain had been felt on the last two occasions, and there was no hæmorrhage, I again used the strong steel pianoforte wire, this time with success, as the tongue was separated just anterior to the epiglottis. There was neither pain nor loss of any blood, and comparatively only little wound to heal; in fact only that part under the tongue which had been cut through within the last three days, for where the base of the tongue had been divided was perfectly healed, shewing, as I suspected, that the separation had been for some time effected there, and that the connections under the tongue are fully sufficient, not only to keep up the vitality of the organ, when its base has been completely divided, and the lingual arteries and nerves severed, but that an enormous crushing force is required to separate the parts. These facts would almost justify suspicion as to the absolute truth of the reports of some few cases in which it is asserted that the whole of the tongue has been removed by a ligature merely carried over its base, which certainly was not effected in this case. The tongue was not in the sloughy condition which might have been anticipated.

"The poor fellow was instantly enabled to talk and swallow with facility. The next day I found him eating a hearty dinner of roast duck, which he declared was the best meal he had taken for more than two years. I now removed the mass of threads and wires which had cut through the tongue, the knots were all firm and well made; one ligature was so firmly planted that I did not remove it until November 15th, when it had to be cut away from near to the cornua of the os-hyoides, and another was so completely buried that it was lost sight of, and only became detached on the 27th, after which the small fistulous opening under the chin immediately closed. The wound in the mouth was cicatrized within two days after the tongue had separated. That there had been no fault in the tying of the ligatures or giving way of the knots, I think these two last-removed threads will prove. All the ligatures had been, except one, placed accurately on the same line; this had caused a small projecting tubercle by partially dividing its connection; I cut it off by a wire ligature.

"The case might be said to be well from the moment the tongue came away; not only was the appetite good, but the power of mastication and swallowing he declared to be much better than they had been for the two previous years. Drinking, as might be anticipated, is more impaired than is the deglutition of solids; indeed, I think few persons would be prepared to find how great a power is enjoyed, and how perfectly the sense of taste remains, while the capability of articulation is considerably beyond expectation. He can pronounce every letter of the alphabet, many of them perfectly (all the vowels), most of them distinctly. The three there is most difficulty in are k, q, and t, which are difficult and indistinct in the order they are named, k being much more so than t. In conversation he can be readily understood, if not excited or hurried. If he be, some words are indistinct, otherwise the power of articulation is sufficient for all purposes of intercourse, so much so, that I believe he will be appointed as master at one of the smaller stations on the railway.

"It will not improbably be thought that much time was unnecessarily taken up, before separation of the tongue was obtained. This is very possible, although I might point to the final success as proof to the contrary, and ask if this very delay was not one means by which success was secured. The loss of a very small additional quantity of blood would, doubtless, have been fatal, and until I felt confident that the danger of this was past, I feared to interfere too much, lest I might provoke it before he had rallied enough to bear what might likely enough follow, had the tongue been removed at an early period, while the tendency to hæmorrhage was great—and the pain caused by the application of the ligatures was so great and exhausting until the nerves were divided, that I wished to avoid it, lest in his weak condition it might turn the scale against him. Yet in another case I should certainly attempt to curtail the time, should circumstances induce a repetition of the same method of proceeding as was adopted in this, by the employment at an earlier period of the strong steel wire ligature, for I do not believe either stronger material or more tightly tied animal or vegetable threads can be used.

"Though well knowing how ineffectual such ligatures are in strangulating a thick portion of the living body, I was not prepared, any more than those friends who kindly assisted me, to suppose that any living tissue could have resisted these repeated applications, made with such force as was used. The employment in the first instance of metallic ligatures of sufficient strength would involve serious difficulty.

"On the other hand, I see no safer means suggested for arresting the hæmorrhage which the use of the knife for the removal of the entire tongue must cause, than the splitting up of the lower jaw, as practised by Mr. Syme. This in itself, as I have said, is very serious, and lays open so large a cavity necessarily exposed to the air, in close proximity with the chest, the patient being, by his inability to swallow and otherwise, unfavourably circumstanced for the treatment of complications, should they arise, that most surgeons will agree with the conclusions of that able operator, as to the inadvisability of having recourse to the knife.

"There remains, then, but the ecraseur, which I should be disposed to employ in another case, in preference to either the ligature or the knife, but I am not sure the operation should be completed at one sitting. It would be a fair subject for consideration, if it might not be more advisable to cut through the base of the tongue by a submental aperture, having, as was done in this case, first divided with the knife all the parts where no serious hæmorrhage is likely to occur, and then to wait for a few hours, or a day, before cutting through the sublingual connections, by which less shock would be caused to the system, than by suddenly crushing through so great an extent of highly vitalized parts at once, as appears to have been done by M. Chassaignac at the Hôpital Levubossière, in Paris. Of course I only speak of cases in which the entire tongue has to be removed, for where even a very large part has to be taken away, there would be no need for the submental aperture, as by the introduction through the substance of the tongue, on each side, of a stout steel needle, the chain of the ecraseur could be fixed far enough back to cut deeply into the organ, so as to crush away at least the two anterior thirds, and thus inflict a much less serious wound than the submental opening must do.

"Thinking the Fellows of the Society present might be interested in seeing the man, I have brought him here to-night, so that an opportunity will be afforded for their personally ascertaining how much less mischief the loss of the tongue inflicts, than perhaps the majority of us would, *à priori*, suppose must be. It is recorded that at least one, if not more, of the early Christian martyrs in Rome continued to speak after the tongue had been torn out, which then, naturally enough, was regarded as a miracle. Such cases as the present will show that, admitting the full truth of the facts, supernatural intervention need not be called in for their explanation.

"Rawlings had some difference with the railway authorities and left their service. He is now keeping a public-house in Wakefield. His speech is greatly improved, and is sufficient for all purposes of intercourse; indeed casual observers would only suppose he had some little impediment in his articulation. "T. N."

On this memoir it is proper to remark that Mr. Nunneley, in being the author of it, becomes an unexceptionable witness to two important points: first, that the whole body of the tongue was removed from Mr. Rawlings; and secondly, that in the same month that the operation was performed he was able to converse intelligibly. In regard to the tongue, the incision was made at the base of that organ just anterior to the hyoid bone. Undoubtedly some portion of the tongue's muscles still adhered to the bone; but I am assured by one of the most eminent living anatomists that unless the hyoid bone were actually scraped, it would be impossible to cut out the tongue more completely.

2. The above is evidence of the operator respecting Mr. Rawlings' loss of his tongue and of his power of speech. What next follows is the evidence on the same two points of Mr. Rawlings, the person operated on. It is contained in a letter which he wrote to me

in February 1862, in answer to one which I had written to him. The questions asked of him may be inferred from his reply.

"Kirkgate, Wakefield, Feb. 22, 1862.

"SIR,—In answer to yours of yesterday, I beg to say, first, I can converse intelligibly with my neighbours, and do so habitually. I can pronounce all vowels and consonants without difficulty, but not so clear since the operation, and I spoke immediately it dropped out into my hand, and my speech has been mending ever since. There is no portion of my tongue left that I am aware of, and I have no difficulty in swallowing; generally the difficulty is in the mouth, that is getting the food into the throat. It is no trouble to answer your questions, and should you wish to ask any more, I will answer them to the best of my ability. I have taken these beer and porter stores, and trust shall be able to make a living with the assistance of my friends, of whom I stand in need, having lost my situation through losing my tongue. Hoping you will remember me,

"I remain, Sir,

"Your most obedient humble Servant,

"ROBERT RAWLINGS."

3. Subsequently, I requested Mr. Rawlings to be good enough to call on me when he came to London;

but I did not receive a visit from him till the following May, when he called on me unexpectedly under circumstances which prevented me from bestowing a concentrated attention on his case. He brought with him in a bottle what he stated to be his own tongue. He opened his mouth wide for inspection, and I could see no tongue in it. At my request he then went through the pronunciation of each of the letters of the alphabet. This he did so distinctly, except as to "d" and "t," that being unwilling to trust only to my own sense of distinguishing sounds, I requested a lady to come to hear him. She did so, and in her hearing he went again through the pronunciation of all the letters of the alphabet with precisely the same distinctness, subject to the same exceptions. I did not specially examine him in particular words; but, generally, he seemed to me to speak with somewhat of an occasional lisp, though every word which he uttered was intelligible. As a memorial of the interview, I took down from his lips the following statement, which was made in answer to my questions :—

"I shall be thirty-six on the 9th of next June. I was born at Cherhill in Wiltshire, near Calne. My father was a farmer at Cherhill. At eighteen I entered the army, in the first battalion of Grenadier Guards. I continued in the army a year and a half, when I paid 20*l.* for my discharge. That was in 1846.

Statement of Mr. Rawlings.

I then went home to my mother at Cherhill (my father being dead), and I remained with her until I married in December 1849. I then was porter and afterwards guard on the London and North-Western Railway. Afterwards I left the railway company, and was a policeman in Staffordshire. Afterwards I was a porter and then an inspector on the Lancashire and Yorkshire Railway, and at last a guard, it being thought that this would benefit my health. At last, on account of the cancer in my tongue, I was obliged to give up my situation altogether. I gave it up last year, about a fortnight before the operation was performed on my tongue.

"I have not suffered in my throat in the slightest degree since the operation was performed. I speak much more clearly now than I did at first. For some time I could not pronounce Q, but I am able to pronounce it now. The letter which I have the greatest difficulty in pronouncing is T. I can pronounce every other letter more easily than T, but I can also pronounce T when I take pains.

"I have a wife and four children. The age of the oldest, a girl, is twelve years and four months; of the next, who is also a girl, ten years; the third is a boy, about three years old; and the youngest is a girl, about fourteen months old. I am still residing at Wakefield, and am keeping beer stores there.

      "ROBERT RAWLINGS."

That others might have an opportunity of seeing Mr. Rawlings and of scrutinizing his case, I requested him to call on several gentlemen whom I named. In one important instance he failed through missing a railway train, and in another instance he failed through some misunderstanding. But he called successively on Sir Charles Lyell, Professor Huxley, Dr. Milman (the late dean of St. Paul's), Professor Owen, and Professor Faraday; and I publish the statements made by each of those eminent men respecting their interviews with him.

4. The following was a minute made by Sir Charles Lyell. It bears date May 20, 1862.

"Mr. Robert Rawlings called on me with an introduction from Mr. Twisleton. Showed me his tongue, preserved in spirits, which had been extracted for cancer.

"He opened his mouth wide that I might see that he had lost the whole of his tongue.

"He said he had been, and still was, suffering from a bad cold and inflammation of the bowels, and that his articulation was not as good as it was when he was not suffering from indisposition.

"He told me that the word 'Leeds' (name of the town) was the one which he found the most difficult to pronounce.

"He repeated all the letters of the alphabet to me

distinctly. In speaking of 'Leeds' he made me at once understand what the word was which it was not easy for him to speak.

"At first he could not pronounce Q, and could only say 'Coo.'

"*Th* somewhat approaches *d* but is intelligible.

"CHARLES LYELL."

5. The following was the statement of Professor Huxley. It was addressed to me in a letter, the greater part of which was written the day after an interview with Mr. Rawlings on the 20th of May, though the letter was not forwarded to its destination till the August following:—

"Sir Charles Lyell some time ago told me that you wished to have my opinion about Mr. Rawlings, the man whose tongue had been excised; and as he called upon me yesterday, I send you the result of my examination, in case you should be in any immediate want of such information as I can supply.

"The man has assuredly lost a very large portion of his tongue, but how much it is not easy to say. When the mouth is wide open, the face of the truncated stump, if I may so call it, of the tongue is on a level with what anatomists call the anterior pillars of the fauces, and Mr. Rawlings told me that as long as his mouth remained open he could advance the stump no further, but that when his mouth was shut, he was able to bring it forwards a good way. The spirit in which the amputated portion of the tongue was placed was so cloudy that no satisfactory examination of its character could be made. On this point, however, Mr. Nunneley, who operated, could doubtless give full information.

"Mr. Rawlings had been ill, and was obviously still indisposed, and he informed me that on this account his speech was by no means so good as usual. However, his words were almost always intelligible, and the majority of them were very fairly pronounced. The only consonants which he was wholly unable to pronounce were *t*'s and *d*'s, initial and final. When initial they were converted into *f, p, v, sh;* when final, they ran into the same letters.

"Thus— tin became fin,
toll „ pool,
tack „ fack, or pack,
dog   „ shog,
dine „ vine,
dew   „ thew,
mad   „ madf,
cat   „ catf.

"Initial *g*'s and *k*'s were well pronounced.

"Final *g*'s were all more or less guttural, like the German *ch*.

"Thus— big became bich (German)
   pig   „   pich.

"*L*'s and *r*'s were slightly imperfect.

"*S*'s, whether initial or final, were imperfect or lisping.

"*Sh* had peculiar difficulties. Such a word as 'shower,' for example, being pronounced in a curious semi-lisping manner, which I know not how to reproduce by our ordinary notation.

"Thus Mr. Rawlings's pronunciation accords pretty well with what might have been predicted from the known mode in which the tongue takes part in the formation of different consonantal sounds.

"*T* and *d* require the tip of the tongue to be brought into contact with the teeth, or quite the anterior part of the palate, and Mr. Rawlings converted them all into *f*'s, *p*'s, *v*'s, or *sh*'s, the apposition of the stump of his tongue to the fore part of the palate being necessarily very imperfect.

"Those consonants again, such as *v* and *z*, for the pronunciation of which it is necessary for the tongue to be in contact with the anterior half of the palate, without very strict occlusion, were given more or less imperfectly.

"Of the sounds which are produced by the combination of the tongue with the posterior part of the palate, on the other hand, Mr. Rawlings was quite master, except final *g*. This I think may be accounted for by the fact that, for a good final *g* the cavity of the back part of the mouth must be completely stopped by the tongue. If the stoppage is incomplete, the sound acquires a guttural prolongation.

"I suppose the stump of the tongue does not fit well.

"On similar grounds, I think we may account for the circumstance that while a good *t* seemed an impossibility to Mr. Rawlings, the *th*'s were very fair.

"Mr. Rawlings was so obviously indisposed that, although he submitted most willingly to my examination, I did not like to keep him more than about half an hour. This period was almost entirely devoted to finding out the defects in his speech, and to the endeavour to discover their precise nature by making him pronounce critical words.

"I am bound to add, therefore, that I conceive it to be quite possible for any person, not on the look-out for difficulties and imperfections, to hold a conversation of some length with Mr. Rawlings without suspecting for a moment the extent of mutilation which he has undergone.

"Listening carelessly, you notice an odd lisping impediment in his speech, like that of a person who has lost part of his palate, and that is all.

"Aug. 8, 1862."

"The greater part of the above account was written

immediately after Mr. Rawlings left me on the 28th of May, 1862, but I thought I would wait until I should see or hear from you before troubling you with it.

"Such as it is, it is very much at your service."

6. Mr. Rawlings called on Dean Milman, at the Deanery, St. Paul's, on Saturday the 14th of June, and I received a letter from the dean in the following week, dated Monday, June 16. The following is the portion of that letter which relates to Mr. Rawlings :—

"The man without a tongue visited and held conversation with me on Saturday. I am much obliged to you for sending him to me. It is a very curious fact. Though I had not the slightest doubt, from what I had heard from trustworthy Oriental travellers, of the credibility of such a case, yet ocular demonstration is always satisfactory. Mr. Rawlings allowed me and even pressed me to look into his throat, and to convince myself of the total extirpation of the tongue, and his speech even to my somewhat imperfect hearing was quite intelligible. Indeed, there were only a few sounds which he could not utter with distinctness. He told me that he had seen Owen (Huxley), who had examined him closely. I shall be curious to hear his commentary on the case."

7. The following was the letter of Professor Owen. It was dated "British Museum, June 21, 1862."

"The faculty of speech is so complete in Mr. Rawlings that, when introduced into my room, I thought it must be some other person from the distinctness of the first remark he made.

"After examining the excised tongue in the bottle of spirits, and the cicatrix adherent to the hyoid bone, I thought that no excision of the tongue could be more complete.

"No doubt, in cases where the tongue was wrenched out by violence, the hyoid and larynx might receive injury, and articulate speech be abrogated.

"My pressing engagements and duties have left me no time for the series of alphabetical observations requisite for a full account of the faculty possessed by the poor remnant of the lingual organ. But Mr. Rawlings's conversation is more easily followed than that of many I have listened to who are affected by nervous stammering."

8. Mr. Rawlings called subsequently on Professor Faraday, who wrote to me the following letter on the subject, dated "The Green, Hampton Court, 19th of August, 1862."

"I saw Mr. Rawlings of Sheffield, and his tongue

(which he had in a bottle), and put him through the sounds of our language as well as I could.

"He spoke wonderfully well—not merely intelligibly, but as well as many persons with their full amount of tongue. If I had not known beforehand that he had lost his tongue, I should not have guessed it from his conversation, though I might have thought his utterance was thick. I put him through the letters of the alphabet, and through syllables and phrases in which the consonants were respectively predominant. There were only one or two sounds in which there was any deficiency, and then not more than in the cases of many persons using their tongues freely. My memory is bad, and I cannot now recal which sounds these were.

"He told me he was in very ill-health when I saw him (and so he seemed to be), and that he could pronounce these sounds much better when he was in health.

"Looking into his mouth, his tongue seemed entirely gone, but I understand that some of the roots remained. Of that I am no judge, but the mouth when open was an empty cavern.

"I waited at the time to see Sir Charles Lyell, but you know what grave circumstances then called him into Italy, and so my communication of the result of the examination to you was interrupted."

I have only to add respecting Mr. Rawlings that the distinctness of his articulation varied somewhat at different times with the state of his health; that his health afterwards entirely failed, and that on the 23rd of February in the following year (1863) he died on a visit to his mother at Church Street, Calne.

11.—*Case attested by Professor Syme.*

In January, 1866, the late Professor Syme, who was thirty-six years Professor of Clinical Surgery in the University of Edinburgh, communicated to the 'Lancet' a case in which a patient spoke distinctly from whom he had removed the whole of the tongue somewhat more than a twelvemonth previously. This case resembled that of Mr. Rawlings in the point that both patients had been suffering from cancer of the tongue. But there was a difference in the mode of operation, for while Mr. Nunneley had made his primary incision between the under jaw and the hyoid bone, Professor Syme (b. 1799, d. 1870), who had twice before operated in the same manner, began by cutting through the under lip, and sawing through the under jaw.

The fact that Professor Syme had removed the whole tongue of his patient had been announced by him in the 'Lancet' of the 14th of February, 1865, and he had given a very clear account of the circumstances which had induced him to undertake the operation. It seems that a Mr. W——, from Manchester, aged 52, had applied to him on account of a form of cancer in the tongue, which not only prevented articulation, but which rendered it impossible for him to swallow solids, and very difficult for him to swallow fluids. It so happened that Professor Syme's two previous cases had terminated unfavourably, and this made him extremely unwilling to repeat the experiment of cutting out the tongue. He therefore suggested palliatives, and recommended his patient to return home. Mr. W—— accordingly returned to Manchester; but his symptoms there becoming aggravated, and death from starvation seeming imminent, he wrote urgently to beg that some form of relief might be devised for him. Under these circumstances, Professor Syme, after giving his patient warning of the very serious danger to life which the operation involved, undertook to remove the whole of the tongue in order to afford him a chance of escape. The patient then returned to Edinburgh, and submitted, on the 29th of December, 1864, to the removal of the whole of his tongue. The fact, and the manner in which it was accomplished, were recorded by Professor Syme in the following words :—

"The operation was performed on the 29th, with the assistance of Mr. Annandale, Dr. Sewell, and Mr. Cheyne, to the first of whom I am especially indebted for his able co-operation. Having extracted one of the front incisors, I cut through the middle of the lip, and continued the incision down to the os-hyoides, then sawed through the jaw in the same line, and insinuating my finger under the tongue as a guide to the knife, divided the mucous lining of the mouth together with the attachment of the genio-hyoglossi. While the two halves of the bone were held apart, I dissected backwards and cut through the hyoglossi along with the mucous membrane covering them, so as to allow the tongue to be pulled forward, and bring into view the situation of the lingual arteries which were cut and tied, first on one side and then on the other. The process might now have been at once completed, had I not feared that the epiglottis might be implicated in the disease, which extended beyond the reach of my finger, and thus suffer injury from the knife if used without a guide. I therefore cut away about two-thirds of the tongue, and then, being able to reach the os-hyoides with my finger, retained it there while the remaining attachments were divided by the knife in my other hand close to the bone. Some small arterial branches having been tied, the edges of the wound were brought together and retained by silver sutures, except at the lowest part, where the ligatures were allowed to maintain a drain for the discharge of fluids from the cavity."

After mentioning some further details, Professor Syme then stated that under an ample supply of nourishment by milk, soup, and solid food, his patient improved in strength so rapidly, that at the end of three weeks he declared he had never felt better in his life. And on the 23rd of January, 1865, within a period of less than four weeks from the date of the operation, he returned to Manchester.

In this first report on the excision of Mr. W——'s tongue, no statement was made as to his subsequent power of articulation. The case was very different in Professor's Syme's second communication to the 'Lancet,' which was published in that journal on the 27th of January, 1866. This report relates that a few months after the removal of the patient's tongue he was able to speak so distinctly that he could enter into conversation with strangers without their discovering the deficiency under which he laboured. Professor Syme took pains to bring the case under the notice of others, and he specifies the course which he adopted with this object. I now reprint the whole of his second report, which will show that the case was thoroughly investigated in a scientific manner, so as to place beyond dispute the fact of the patient's distinct articulation.

"About twelve months ago I communicated a case in which the tongue had been completely removed by excision, on account of extensive disease that threatened to prove fatal by preventing the admission of nourishment. This account was necessarily limited to the operation and its immediate effects, as sufficient time had not elapsed for determining whether or no the relief afforded would prove permanent, or how far the powers of deglutition, articulation, and taste would be restored. After his return home to Manchester, the patient sent me favourable reports of his progress, but certainly not such as to convey any adequate idea of the improvement that had taken place since he came under my care. He was then emaciated and bent down by long-continued suffering, unable to articulate, so as to require a slate and pencil for expressing his wishes, and swallowing even fluids with such extreme difficulty as to feel on the point of starvation. My surprise may therefore be imagined when on the 10th of September last he unexpectedly made his appearance erect and vigorous, and seeing that I did not recognize him, announcing his name in a loud clear voice. The feeling thus excited was not lessened by learning that while travelling in the Highlands he had dined at table d'hôtes, and entered into conversation without betraying the deficiency under which he laboured. Very much astonished by a result so much better than could have been anticipated, I requested a number of my medical friends to join me in examining the state of matters. Professor Goodsir and Mr. Nasmyth having satisfied themselves that no vestige of the tongue remained, various observations were made with regard to articulation, and other functions of the absent organ: and Mr. Annandale afterwards instituted a more particular inquiry, of which he has given me the following report:—

"'The lips and jaw-bone, where divided, were soundly united without any deformity. The opening between the mouth and pharynx was much diminished in size and irregular in shape from contraction of the fauces and soft palate, which were drawn downwards and forwards more to the right than the left side, from the mucous membrane at that part having participated in the disease and been removed along with the tongue. Mr. W—— says that he can swallow as well as ever, provided that the food is either finely divided or fluid. He is also able to masticate solid substances, although difficulty is sometimes experienced from their getting into awkward parts of the mouth. In ordinary speech his words are wonderfully clear and distinct, and he can sing without any difficulty. All the vowels and words composed of them are articulated perfectly, and also the following consonants: B, C, F, H, K, L, M, N, P, Q, R, V, W. D is pronounced "dthe;" J, "the;" G, like "sjee." S is a lisp. His taste is impaired, but still enables him to distinguish different articles and their respective qualities, as grouse from partridge, bitters from sweets, good beer from bad beer, &c. He has remarked that the seat of sensation lies somewhere in the throat, since there is no recognition of taste previous to the act of swallowing; and in order to ascertain the truth of this point more precisely, the following experiments were made:—

"'1. A strong solution of salt was applied by means of a camel-hair brush to the fauces, palate, floor of the mouth, lips, and inner surface of the cheek, with the result of something being felt in the mouth, but no idea formed as to its nature.

"'2. About a quarter of a teaspoonful of finely-powdered sugar was placed on the floor of the mouth, and having been allowed to remain there a few seconds was then brought thoroughly into contact with every part of the cavity without any recognition of its nature; but when a little water was added and swallowed, the taste was immediately perceived.

"'3. The same experiment was repeated with another substance (salt), and with the same result.

"'It has long been known that large portions of the tongue may be removed without destroying or materially impairing the power of articulation; but I am not aware of any case on record in which it has remained so perfect after complete removal of the organ. Of the facts above mentioned, the one that seems most curious is the connexion between taste and deglutition; from which it appears that the latter is essential for the full perception of the former. If the pleasure of taste could be perfectly gratified by mastication without deglutition, there would be no limit to the consumption of food; but the instinctive desire to swallow an agreeable morsel affords a check to any such abuse.

"'As the nature of the disease was not particularly described in relating the operation, a representation of the microscopic structure exhibited by the tumour (for which I am indebted to Mr. Annandale) may be given to shew that it possessed the characters of epithelial cancer.'"

12.—*Cases attested by Sir James Paget.*

While this work was in preparation it occurred to me as desirable to ascertain from Sir James Paget, the very distinguished surgeon, whether any case of a person's speaking although his tongue had been cut off had come within his own observation. The result of my inquiries on this point is that Sir James has known no less than six such cases, in which he himself had removed a large portion of the tongue. After the evidence already produced, it seems unnecessary to enter into very minute details on each of these cases, but the name and address of each of the persons operated on can, if he is still alive, be procured without great difficulty. At the same time the following statement of Sir James Paget, which he has had the kindness to write to me, is sufficient to remove any doubt as to the reality of there having been six such cases within his own knowledge. Sir James Paget states as follows :—

"I have six times removed what is commonly spoken of as the whole tongue—*i.e.*, as much as can be drawn out of the mouth after separating the attachments of the tongue to the lower jaw. This includes the whole length of the tongue to within a quarter of an inch of the arches of the palate, and its thickness to the level of the floor of the mouth, a much larger portion, I believe, than is removed in any of the instances of cutting out the tongue as a punishment.

"All the patients thus operated on could talk quickly and intelligibly after the healing of their wounds. Of course they could not pronounce the sounds requiring the tip of the tongue—as t, d, th—but the absence of these sounds did not make their speech more unclear than that of persons who lisp, or who use w for r, or ph for th.

"They could speak intelligibly, though not very clearly, soon after the operation. One patient, directly after waking from the influence of chloroform, said plainly, 'God bless you.' Another, on the day after the operation, said, so that all around understood him, 'I should like some cold brandy and water.' But I think that, generally, the speech was less clear a few days after the operation; probably because of the swelling of the parts about the wound. With the subsidence of the swelling, and the healing of the wound, the speech became constantly more distinct.

"There is no truth in the statement that speech is destroyed by the removal of the tip of the tongue. Speech is less affected by this operation than by the removal of large portions of the side. I have only once performed the operation for cancer: for this disease is very rarely seated in the tip of the tongue alone. In that case, the speech was scarcely perceptibly affected. In hypertrophy or overgrowth of the tongue, in which all the foretop or tip becomes enormous, removal of the part does not materially affect the speech. I have twice performed this operation, and both patients talked well after it. The tip of the tongue has also been bitten off in falls on the lower jaw: and I have never heard of such an accident being followed by loss or serious impediment of speech. I have very often spoken on the subject with surgeons who have had large experience in operations on the tongue, and I have never heard of a case in which the removal of any portion, or the whole, of the tongue was followed by loss of the power of speech."

It only remains to observe that the facts last mentioned by Sir James Paget are conclusive to prove that loss of the power of speech is not the necessary consequence of cutting off the mere tip of the tongue. It seems equally certain that a contrary idea prevails in the East, and that individuals there have been so disabled from speech by the excision of the tip of the tongue, that they have submitted to a second operation for the removal of the whole of that portion of the tongue which is loose in the mouth. There are no decisive data for explaining this last class of facts. Perhaps an explanation may be found in the suggestion that Eastern executioners from a fear of being punished for not having done their work properly, if their victims were able to speak immediately, or from hopes of pecuniary gain, through being called upon to perform a second operation, may practise mangling the tip of the tongue in their first operation so as to disable it from speech. Sir James Paget himself is in favour of this explanation, and he makes a further statement as follows:—"I believe that the tip of a tongue may be so mangled as to make speaking very difficult and painful for a time, and till the mangled part either heals or sloughs away. During this time, or for at least one or two days after the mangling, speaking would be made easier by cutting off the mangled part." And this explanation precisely tallies with the statement of Mehdee Kooly Beg, above recorded in page 118, that he was speechless after the tip of his tongue was cut off. For it will be observed that the Persian executioner had previously claimed fifty tomauns (25*l.*) "to perform the operation well," and that Mehdee Kooly had refused to give that sum, before he submitted his tongue to be operated on by the executioner.

V.

CONCLUSION.

NUMEROUS cases, all attested by some direct evidence have now been adduced, which bear more or less on the supposed miraculous power of speech in the African confessors. The following points may be mentioned as a summary of results from that evidence.

1. The tongue is not indispensable for purposes of speech. A general impression has prevailed that the tongue is the organ of speech in the same sense that the ear is the organ of hearing and the eye is the organ of sight. But this is a mistake. Some persons have been known to speak intelligibly with the tip of the tongue cut off, some with all that is loose in the mouth cut off, some with a still larger portion cut off, and some with the whole body of the tongue cut out. A boy spoke intelligibly who lost his tongue from gangrene when he was eight or nine years old, and two young women spoke intelligibly, of whom one had lost her tongue from cancer when

Conclusion.

four years old, and the other was born without any tongue at all.

2. It is an impossible operation to cut out the whole tongue simply through the ordinary aperture of the mouth. The only instances on record in which the whole tongue has been cut out from living persons are cases in which previously either the under jaw was sawn through, or an incision had been made between the chin and the hyoid bone. And these cases are of very recent date.

3. It may be regarded as reasonably certain that the tongues of the African confessors were cut out solely through the ordinary aperture of the mouth. Their punishment was inflicted on them publicly in the Forum of Tipasa. It is unlikely that in 484 there was sufficient surgical knowledge to enable an operator, without death to the victim, to cut out the tongue by aid of an incision under the chin, or by sawing through the under-jaw. If there had been such surgical knowledge, the operation could not have been effected publicly on many persons on the same day. And if any such operation had taken place the fact would have undoubtedly been mentioned by Victor Vitensis or others, in aggravation of the atrocity of the punishment.

4. The statements made by a long series of writers, beginning with the eye-witnesses, Victor Vitensis and Æneas of Gaza, that the tongues of the confessors

were cut out or torn out by the roots, and the consequent expressions that the confessors spoke without tongues must be regarded as inaccurate.* This inaccuracy is now unimportant in reference to the miraculousness of their speech, for there is evidence which shows that they might possibly have spoken as well without tongues as they spoke with mutilated tongues. Still, in reference to the strict facts of the case the expressions used on this point were inaccurate. Indeed, previous to Sir John McNeill, no writer seems to have conceived rightly the result of the punishment, and to have been aware that the sufferers still possessed a portion of their tongues, however mutilated, after the executioner had done his worst. This is a remarkable instance that in matters of this kind even honest eye-witnesses cannot always be depended on, unless they have sound special knowledge, inasmuch as they may easily mislead by importing into their statements their own pre-conceived ideas.

* When I published an article on the confessors in 'Notes and Queries,' in 1858, I was under the erroneous impression that the retention by the confessors of a portion of their tongues was a point of importance in reference to the supposed miracle. I had not then read the treatise of M. Roland on the Saumur case, the report of M. Jussieu on the Portuguese case, or the reports on the case of Margaret Cutting in the 'Transactions' of the Royal Society.

Conclusion.

5. The great preponderance of evidence is in favour of the supposition that in persons with mutilated tongues or without tongues, there is likely to be some slight defect in the pronunciation of some letters in words, especially of "d" and "t." In regard to the confessors, there is no detailed information on this point, as no attempt seems to have been made to test their pronunciation of particular letters or words. The general expressions, indeed, respecting the distinctness of their articulation, are very strong. Among the eye-witnesses and ear-witnesses, Victor Vitensis says, "they spoke as well as they spoke before," and of Reparatus he says that he spoke "without any impediment." Æneas of Gaza goes beyond Victor Vitensis, and says the confessors spoke articulately and *better* than before. Moreover Count Marcellinus and Procopius both say that the confessors spoke with an entire, unimpaired, or perfect voice; the Latin word "integrâ," used by Marcellinus (from which our own word "entire" is derived through the French), being precisely equivalent in this passage to the Greek word used by Procopius.[b] Still these statements

---

[b] Grotius in his Latin version of Procopius on the Vandal war correctly translates ἀκραιφνής by "integer." His rendering of the words in Procopius ('De Bell. Vand.' i. 8). ἐχρῶντο ἀκραιφνεῖ τῇ φωνῇ, is "*integro* utentes sermone." The translation in the Bonn edition of 1833, "*explanatè* loquebantur," is less good. See Grotius, 'Historia Gotthorum, Vandalorum,' &c. Amstelodami, 1655.

must not be pressed so far as to be deemed incompatible with a slightly defective pronunciation of certain letters. Possibly, if M. Jussieu, or Professor Huxley, or Sir James Paget had examined the confessors closely and scientifically, it would have been perceived that their pronunciation of "d" and "t," and perhaps of some other letters was not wholly faultless. It is true that Dr. Tulp in his observations on the case of Joannes the Dumb, whose tongue had been mutilated by Turkish pirates, uses expressions absolutely identical with those of Marcellinus, Procopius, and Æneas of Gaza. Dr. Tulp speaks with wonder of Joannes's voice as having come back entirely, or in a perfect state (vocem *integrè* rediisse). Moreover, he says that Joannes uttered his words very articulately; and that he not only spoke distinctly, but "pronounced accurately all the consonants, the utterance of which had usually been attributed to the tip of the tongue alone."[e] But that a general description of a voice as "perfect" is not necessarily incompatible with some slight defect in its articulation

---

[e] See Appendix E. Mr. Rawlings pronounced successively the individual letters of the alphabet so well that it would be unsafe to assert positively that Joannes could not have pronounced them *perfectly* well. The pronunciation of separate letters must be carefully distinguished from the pronunciation of whole words, which is a matter of greater difficulty.

of some letters is shown conclusively by expressions made use of by Dr. Parsons. For in one part of his Report on Margaret Cutting, he states "her voice is perfect;" and yet in another part he admits a defect in her pronunciation of the five apex letters; though he adds that "those she manages so well by bringing the under lip to her upper teeth in the course of her conversation that any one can instantly apprehend every word she says." And Mr. Boddington, Mr. Notcutt, and Mr. Hammond had previously, without any qualification, spoken of her as pronouncing even those apex letters "perfectly."

The final result seems to be that questions connected with the phenomenon of speech in the African confessors are purely within the domain of natural science, and that there is no reason for asserting or suspecting any miraculous intervention in the matter. It is true that their tongues were mutilated by a tyrant for illegal conduct, which sprang solely from zeal for their religion; but this does not tend to render their speech miraculous. It would be equally reasonable to regard as miraculous all cases of Protestant confessors, who, having been cruelly tortured by Roman Catholic inquisitors, escaped with their lives; although it were shown that others had escaped with their lives from precisely the same tortures, when religion had been neither the cause nor the pretext of their punishment.

APPENDIX A.

THE ORIGINAL AUTHORITIES FOR THE HISTORY OF THE AFRICAN CONFESSORS.

In order to save the trouble of referring to eight different works, the original passages are here collected together, in which the following eight persons advert to the case of the African Confessors, viz.—

1. Victor Vitensis.
2. Æneas of Gaza.
3. Procopius of Cæsareia.
4. The Emperor Justinian.
5. Count Marcellinus.
6. Victor Tunonensis.
7. Pope Gregory the First.
8. Isidore, Archbishop of Seville.

From the 'Historia Persecutionis Vandalicæ,' by Victor Vitensis. Lib. v. c. 6.

In Typasensi vero quod gestum est Mauritaniæ majoris civitate ad laudem Dei insinuare festinemus. Dum suæ civitati Arianum episcopum ex notario Cyrilæ ad perdendas animas ordinatum vidissent, omnis simul civitas evectione navali de proximo ad Hispaniam confugit, relictis paucissimis, qui aditum non invenerant navigandi. Quos Arianorum episcopus primo blandimentis, postea minis compellere cœpit, ut eos faceret Arianos. Sed fortes in Domino permanentes, non solum suadentis insaniam irrisêrunt; verum etiam publicè mysteria divina in domo unâ congregati celebrare cœpêrunt. Quod ille cognoscens, relationem occulte Carthaginem adversus eos direxit; quæ cum regi innotuisset, comitem quemdam cum iracundiâ dirigens, præcepit ut in medio foro congregatâ illuc omni provinciâ, linguas eis et manus dexteras radicitus abscidisset. Quod cum factum fuisset, Spiritu Sancto præstante, ita locuti sunt et loquuntur, quomodo antea loquebantur. Sed si quis incredulus esse voluerit, pergat nunc Constantinopolim, et ibi reperiet unum de illis, subdiaconem Reparatum, sermones politos sine ullâ offensione loquentem. Ob quam causam venerabilis nimium in palatio Zenonis imperatoris habetur, et præcipue regina mirâ cum reverentiâ veneratur.

From the 'Theophrastus' of Æneas of Gaza.

Τὴν μεγάλην Λιβύην πικρὰ κατέχει τυραννίς. Ἄπιστον δὲ τυραννίδι φιλανθρωπία καὶ ἀληθεῖς δόξαι· ὁ γοῦν τύραννος ἔγκλημα ποιεῖται τὴν τῶν ἀρχομένων εὐσέβειαν, καὶ τοῦτο καλὸν δόγμα τοὺς ἱερέας ἀρνεῖσθαι κελεύει· οὐ πειθομένων δὲ (ὢ τῆς ἀσεβείας) Θεοφιλῆ γλῶτταν ἐκτέμνει. Καθάπερ ὁ τοῦ μύθου Τηρεύς, βεβιασμένης παρθένου, προανελεῖν κατηγορίαν οἰόμενος, τὴν γλῶτταν ἀπέκειρεν. Ἀλλ' ἡ μὲν κόρη ἐνυφαίνει τῷ πέπλῳ τὸ δρᾶμα, καὶ ἑρμηνεύει τῇ τέχνῃ· οὐ γὰρ ἔτι λαλεῖν παρέσχεν ἡ φύσις. Οἱ δὲ πέπλου καὶ τέχνης οὐδὲν δεηθέντες, τὸν τῆς φύσεως, καλοῦσι Δημιουργόν· ὁ δὲ νεωτέραν αὐτοῖς φύσιν ἡμέρᾳ τρίτῃ χαρίζεται· οὐ γλῶτταν ἑτέραν διδούς, ἀλλ' ἄνευ γλώττης σαφέστερον ἢ πρότερον διαλέγεσθαι. Ἐγὼ δὲ ἐπειθόμην ὡς ἀδύνατον αὐλητὴν ἐν ἀπορίᾳ τῶν αὐλῶν αὐλητικὴν ἐπιδείκνυσθαι· ἀδύνατον δὲ κιθαρῳδὸν ἐν ἀπορίᾳ τῆς κιθάρας, μουσικὴν ἐργάζεσθαι· νῦν δέ με τουτὶ τὸ καινὸν θέαμα ἀναγκάζει μετανοεῖν, καὶ μηδὲν τῶν ὁρωμένων πεπηγέναι νομίζειν, εἰ Θεὸς ἐθέλει μετακινεῖν. Εἶδον ἔγωγε τοὺς ἄνδρας, καὶ λαλούντων ἤκουσα, καὶ τῆς φωνῆς τὸ ἔναρθρον θαυμάζων, τὸ τῆς φωνῆς ὄργανον ἐζήτουν· καὶ τοῖς ὠσὶν ἀπιστῶν, τοῖς ὀφθαλμοῖς ἐπέτρεπον τὴν κρίσιν, καὶ τὸ στόμα διανοίγων ὅλην ἐκ ριζῶν ἀνασπασθεῖσαν ἐθεώρουν τὴν γλῶτταν· καὶ ἐκπλαγεὶς ἐθαύμαζον οὐκ ὅπως τὸν λόγον συνήρμοσαν, ἀλλ' ὅπως ἐσώθησαν.—From Migne's '*Patrologiæ Cursus Completus*,' Series Græca, vol. 85.

Extract from Procopius.

Γέγονε δὲ Ὀνώριχος ἐς τοὺς ἐν Λιβύῃ Χριστιανοὺς ὠμότατός τε καὶ ἀδικώτατος ἀνθρώπων ἁπάντων. Βιαζόμενος γὰρ αὐτοὺς ἐς τὴν Ἀριανῶν μετατίθεσθαι δόξαν, ὅσους ἂν λάβοι οὐχ' ἑτοίμους αὐτῷ εἴκοντας, ἔκαιέ τε καὶ ἄλλαις θανάτου ἰδέαις διέφθειρε, πολλῶν δὲ καὶ τὰς γλώσσας ἀπέτεμεν ἀπ' αὐτῆς φάρυγγος, οἳ ἔτι καὶ ἐς ἐμὲ περιόντες ἐν Βυζαντίῳ ἐχρῶντο ἀκραιφνεῖ τῇ φωνῇ, οὐδ' ὁπωστιοῦν ταύτης δὴ τῆς τιμωρίας ἐπαισθανόμενοι· ὧν δὴ δύο, ἐπειδὴ γυναιξὶν ἑταίραις πλησιάζειν ἔγνωσαν, οὐκέτι φθέγγεσθαι τὸ λοιπὸν ἴσχυσαν· ἔτη τε ὀκτὼ Βανδίλων ἄρξας ἐτελεύτησε νόσῳ, κ.τ.λ.—Procopius '*de Bello Vandalico*,' i. 8.

Migne, '*Patrologiæ Cursus Completus*,' vol. 51.
Marcellini '*Chronicon*,' p. 934.
A.C. 484, Ind. VII. *Theodorico et Venantio Coss.*

Illus natione Isaurus, dignitate magister officiorum, amputatâ apud comitatum auriculâ, Orientem Zenoni infestus invasit. Porro, cum Leontio tyrannidem arripuit. Totam namque per Africam crudelis Hunerici Wandalorum regis in nostros catholicos persecutio importata est. Nam exsulatis diffugatisque plusquam CCCXXXIIII. (Chiffl. CCCXXXIII.)

orthodoxorum episcopis ecclesiisque eorum clausis, plebs fidelium, variis subacta suppliciis, beatum consummavit agonem. Nempe tunc idem rex Hunericus, unius Catholici adolescentis vitam a nativitate suâ sine ullo sermone ducentis linguam præcepit excidi idemque mutus quod sine humano auditu Christo credens fide didicerat mox præcisâ sibi linguâ locutus est, gloriamque Deo in primo vocis suæ exordio dedit. Denique ex hoc fidelium contubernio aliquantos ego religiosissimos viros præcisis linguis, manibus truncatis, apud Byzantium integrâ voce conspexi loquentum. Hæc Arianorum crudelitas in religiosos Christi cultores, suprascriptis consulibus mense Februario cœpit infligi.

Edict of the Emperor Justinian in the Justinian Code.

Tit. xxvii.—*De officio Præfecti Prætorio Africæ et de omni ejusdem Diœceseos statu. De judiciis civilium administrationum et officiis eorum.*

Imperator Cæsar Flavius Justinianus, &c., Archelao Præfecto Prætorio Africæ.

Quas gratias aut quas laudes Domino Deo nostro Jesu Christo exhibere debeamus, nec mens nostra potest concipere nec lingua proferre. Multas quidem et antea a Deo meruimus largitates, et innumerabilia circa nos ejus beneficia confitemur, pro quibus nihil dignum nos egisse cognoscimus. Præ omnibus tamen hoc, quod nunc Omnipotens Deus per nos pro suâ laude et pro suo nomine demonstrare dignatus est, excedit omnia mirabilia opera quæ in sæcula contigêrunt, ut Africa per nos tam brevi tempore reciperet libertatem, antea nonaginta quinque annos a Vandalis captivata : qui animarum fuerant simul hostes et corporum: nam animas quidem diversa tormenta atque supplicia non ferentes, rebaptizando, ad suam perfidiam transferebant: corpora vero liberis natalibus clara jugo barbarico durissimè subjugabant: ipsas quoque Dei sacrosanctas Ecclesias suis perfidiis maculabant: aliquas vero ex eis stabula fecêrunt. Vidimus venerabiles viros, qui abscissis radicitus linguis suas pœnas miserabiliter loquebantur. Alii vero post diversa tormenta per diversas dispersi provincias vitam in exilio peragebant. Quo ergo sermone, aut quibus operibus dignas Deo gratias agere valeamus, &c. &c.

Extract from the 'Chronicon' of Victor Tunonensis.

Zenone Aug. Cos., Hunnericus Vandalorum Rex persecutioni per totam Africam nimis insistens, Tubunnis, Macri Nippis, aliisque Eremi partibus Catholicos jam non solum Sacerdotes et cuncti ordinis Clericos, sed et Monachos atque Laicos quatuor circiter millia exiliis durioribus relegat, et Confessores ac Martyres facit, Confessoribusque linguas abscidit. Quos Confessores quod linguis abscissis perfectè finem adusque locuti sunt, Urbs Regia adtestatur, ubi eorum corpora jacent.—*Scaliger's edition of 'Thesaurus Temporum Eusebii Pamphili.'* Amstelodami, 1658, p. 4, i.

Extract from 'Dialogues' of Pope Gregory the First.

Caput xxxii.—*De Episcopis Africanis, qui pro defensione catholicæ fidei, abscissâ ab Arianis Vandalis linguâ, nullum locutionis solitæ sustinuêre dispendium.*

Gregorius.—Justiniani quoque Augusti temporibus dum contra catholicorum fidem exorta a Vandalis persecutio Ariana in Africâ vehementer insaniret, quidam in defensione veritatis episcopi fortiter persistentes, ad medium sunt deducti. Quos Vandalorum rex, verbis ac muneribus ad perfidiam flectere non valens, tormentis frangere posse se credidit. Nam cum eis in ipsâ defensione veritatis silentium indiceret, nec tamen ipsi contra perfidiam tacerent, ne tacendo forsitan consensisse viderentur, raptus in furorem eorum linguas abscidi radicitus fecit. Res mira et multis nota senioribus, quia ita post pro defensione veritatis etiam sine linguâ loquebantur, sicut prius loqui per linguam consueverant.

Petrus.—Mirandum valde et vehementer stupendum.

Gregorius.—Scriptum, Petre, est de Unigenito summi Patris: *In principio erat Verbum, et Verbum erat apud Deum, et Deus erat Verbum* (Joann. i. 1). De cujus etiam virtute subjungitur; *Omnia per ipsum facta sunt (Ibid.).* Quid igitur miramur, si verba edere sine linguâ potuit Verbum quod fecit linguam?

Petrus.—Placet quod dicis.

Gregorius.—Hi itaque, eo tempore profugi, ad Constantinopolitanam Urbem venêrunt. Eo quoque tempore quo pro explendis responsis Ecclesiæ ad Principem ipsum transmissus sum, seniorem quemdam episcopum reperi qui se adhuc eorum ora sine linguis loquentia vidisse testabatur, ita ut apertis oribus clamarent: Ecce videte, quia linguas non habemus et loquimur. Videbatur enim a respicientibus, ut ferebat, quia abscissis radicitus linguis, quasi quoddam barathrum patebat in gutture, et tamen ore vacuo plena ad integrum verba formabantur. Quorum illic unus in luxuriam lapsus, mox privatus est dono miraculi; recto videlicet omnipotentis Dei judicio, ut qui carnis continentiam servare neglexerat, sine linguâ carneâ non haberet verba virtutis. Sed hæc nos pro Arianæ hæreseos damnatione dixisse sufficiat, nunc ad ea quæ nuper in Italiâ gesta sunt signa redeamus.

Isidori Chronicon.

Post Gessericum Unericus Gunderici filius regnat annos septem menses quinque, habens in conjugio Valentiniani filiam, quam pater ejus ex Româ cum matre captivam adduxerat ; qui et ipse Arriano suscitatus furore Catholicos per totam Africam atrocior patre persequitur. Ecclesias tollit, sacerdotes (et cunctos) sacri ordinis clericos exilio mittit. Monachos quoque atque laicos quatuor circiter millia exiliis durioribus relegavit. Martyres fecit, confessoribus linguas abscidit, qui linguis abscissis perfectè usque ad finem locuti sunt. Tunc Lætus, Neptensis civitatis Episcopus (gloriosè martyrio coronatur, qui dum Arriani) contagii labe variis poenis maculari non potuit, victor repentè coelos obtinuit. Unericus autem inter innumerabiles suarum impietatum strages quas in Catholicos exercuerat, octavo regni anno, ut Arrius pater ejus, interioribus cunctis effusis miserabiliter vitam finivit. — From '*Historia Gotthorum Vandalorum et Langobardorum ab Hugone Grotio partim versa, partim in ordinem digesta.*' Amstelodami, 1655.

APPENDIX B.

DR. NEWMAN'S REMARKS ON THE EVIDENCE.

From Dr. Newman's Two Essays on Scripture Miracles and on Ecclesiastical, pp. 381-385. London, 1870.

ONE of the striking points then in this miracle, as contained in the foregoing evidence, is obviously its *completeness*. We know that even deaf and dumb persons can be made in some sense to utter words; and there may be attempts far superior to theirs, yet wanting in that ease and precision which characterize the ordinary gift of speech. But the articulateness, nay, the educated accent of these confessors, is especially insisted on in the testimony. "A cure left thus imperfect," says Douglas, speaking of a Jansenist miracle, "has but little pretension to be looked upon as miraculous, because its being so imperfect naturally points out a failure of power in the cause which brought it about." Whatever be the truth of this position, it cannot be applied to the miracle under review.

The *number* on which it was wrought is another most important circumstance, distinguishing this history from others of a miraculous character. It both increases opportunities for testimony, and it prevents the interposition of what is commonly called chance, which could not operate upon many persons at once in one and the same way. This is the proper answer to Middleton's objection, that cases are on record of speech without a tongue, when no special intervention of Providence could be supposed. Not to say that a person *born* without a tongue, as in the instance to which he refers, may more easily be supposed to have found a compensation for her defect by a natural provision or guidance than men who had ever spoken by the ordinary organ till they came suddenly to lose it. "If we should allow after all," says he, "that the tongues of these confessors were cut away to the very roots, what will the learned doctor (Berriman) say if this boasted miracle which he so strenuously defends, should be found at last to be no miracle at all? The tongue, indeed, has generally been considered as absolutely necessary to the use of speech; so that to hear men talk without it might easily pass for a miracle in that credulous age." And then he mentions the case of a girl born without a tongue, who yet talked as distinctly and easily as if she had enjoyed the full benefit of that organ, according to the report of a French physician who had carefully examined her mouth and throat, and who refers at the same time to another instance, published about eighty years before, of a boy who at the age of eight or nine years lost his tongue by an ulcer after the small-pox, yet retained his speech, whether as perfectly as before does not appear.

Now, taking these instances at their greatest force, does he mean to say that if a certain number of men lost their tongues at the command of a tyrant for the sake of their religion, and then spoke as plainly as before; nay, if only one person was so mutilated and so gifted, it would not be a miracle? if not, why does he not believe the history of these confessors? At least, he might believe that some of them had the gift of speech continued to them, though the numbers be an exaggeration. It is his canon, as Douglas assures us, that while the history of miracles is "to be suspected always of course, without the strongest evidence to confirm it," the history of common events is to be "*admitted of course*, without as strong reason to suspect it." Now, here all the reason or evidence is on the side of believing: yet he does not believe it, why? simply, because as common sense tells us, and as he feels, it *is* a miraculous story. It is far more difficult to believe that a number of men were forbidden to profess orthodoxy, did continue to profess it, were brought into the forum, had their tongues cut out from the roots, survived it, and spoke ever afterwards as they did before, *without* a miracle, than *with* it. But Middleton would secure two weapons at once for his warfare against the claims of the Catholic Church: it *is* a miracle, and therefore it is incredible as a fact; it is *not* a miracle, and therefore it is irrelevant as an argument.

Another remarkable peculiarity of this miracle is what may be called its *entireness*, by which I mean that it carried its whole case with it to every beholder. When a blind man has been restored to sight, there must be one witness to prove he *has been* blind, and another that he *now sees;* when a cure has been effected, we need a third to assure us that no medicines were administered to the subject of it; but here the miracle is condensed in the fact that there is no tongue, and yet a voice. The function of witnessing is far narrower and more definite, yet more perfect, than in other cases.

A further characteristic of this miracle is its *permanence;* and in this respect it throws light upon a remark made in a former page to account for the deficiency of evidence which generally attaches to the ecclesiastical miracles. It was there observed that they commonly took place without notice beforehand, and left no trace after them; and we could not have better or fuller testimony than that which happened to be found on the spot where they occurred. The instance before us, however, being of a permanent character, and carrying its miraculousness in the very sight of it, admitted of its being witnessed in a higher way, and so it is witnessed. Supposing the miracles of St. Gregory Thaumaturgus or St. Martin to have had advantage of similar publicity, at least they would have been disengaged from the misstatements and exaggerations which at present prejudice them, are we sure they would not have gained, instead, a body of testimony to their substantial truth?

APPENDIX C.

FRENCH PROTESTANT MARTYRS.

THE earliest cases in modern times of speech with mutilated tongues, recorded by a contemporary, though not by an eyewitness, seem to be those of some French Protestant Martyrs, whose tongues had been cut off before they were led to the place of execution to be burned alive.

These cases are mentioned by Jean Crespin (— d. 1572), a French advocate connected with the Parliament of Paris, who had adopted the Reformed faith, and had taken refuge in Geneva, where he established a printing press. They are contained in a work published by him at Geneva in 1556, entitled 'Collected Accounts of several persons who have endured death with constancy for the name of the Lord since John Wickliff to the present time.'* He printed this work with his name in the title-page.

One case is that of Etienne Mangin, of Meaux, in whose house fourteen Protestants had been arrested for having met there to celebrate the Lord's Supper. By a sentence at Paris, dated the 4th of October, 1546, Mangin and his companions were all condemned to be burned alive. They

---

* Recueil de plusieurs personnes qui ont constamment enduré la mort pour le nom de Dieu, depuis Jean Wickliffe jusqu'au temps présent. Par Jean Crespin. 1556.

were all submitted to the torture on the 6th of that month. The following day was the day appointed for their execution, and it had been ordered that the tongues of all of them should be cut off before they were led to the stake, with an exception made in favour of those who would consent to be confessed. Eight accepted this condition, but six refused it. Crespin says, generally, of these six that "they did not cease to praise God," nor the others to chant Psalms. But of Mangin he writes specially, as follows: " At the hour of execution, which was about two o'clock in the afternoon, as they were leaving the prison, the executioner first demanded the tongue of Etienne Mangin, who put his tongue wide out voluntarily; and after the executioner had cut it, while spitting blood he still spoke sufficiently intelligibly, saying three times, ' God's name be blessed' (Le nom de Dieu soit béni)."

The other case is that of Gabriel Beraudin, a native of Lodun, who, in April 1550, had been condemned to be burned alive at Chambéry, with Jean Godeau, a native of Chinon. From terror at the prospect of such a death, Beraudin had been induced to retract. On this account his life was to be spared; but he was condemned to make a public atonement for his supposed heresy, and then to be sent to the galleys. In pursuance of his commuted sentence, he was compelled, with nothing on but his shirt, to follow Godeau to the stake, to witness the death of his companion. But in following Godeau, Beraudin was so struck by Godeau's cheerfulness and constancy of mind, that he became ashamed of his own previous weakness; and he retracted his retractation, though he knew what awaited him. He was then led back to prison, and not long after, he was, like Godeau, burned alive. His tongue had been previously cut off; but yet, says Crespin, "in consequence of his holy fervour he did not cease to speak sufficiently intelligibly, so that the provost, in leading the holy martyr to his last punishment, taxed the executioner with not having sufficiently cut the tongue. But the executioner said to him in the presence of many hearers, 'Can I prevent him from speaking?'"

Crespin does not give his authority for these two histories; but, as an advocate attached to the parliament of Paris, he was likely to know what passed when the fourteen Protestants were burned alive at Meaux, and, as a Protestant residing in a time of persecution at Geneva, he was likely to know what passed when Beraudin was burned alive in a town so little distant as Chambéry. Moreover, he published his book not more than six years after the martyrdom of Beraudin, and within ten years after the martyrdom of Mangin. It is to be observed also that Crespin uses scrupulously measured language in reference to the speech both of Mangin and of Beraudin. He merely states of each that he spoke " sufficiently intelligibly;" and he makes no attempt to swell the fact into a miracle. Thus, considering all the cases already recorded in this volume, there does not seem to be any valid reason to doubt the accuracy of Crespin's statements on this subject.

It may be useful, at the same time, to point out that the punishment inflicted on the French martyrs of Meaux was much more cruel than the punishment inflicted by Huneric the Vandal on the African confessors of Tipasa. The African confessors were sentenced to lose their tongues and right hands, but their lives were spared. The French martyrs were tortured and burned alive, and six of them had, likewise, their tongues cut off when led out to execution.

APPENDIX D.

EXTRACT FROM M. ROLAND'S FRENCH WORK,
'*Aglossostomographie; ou, Description d'une Bouche sans Langue.*' Saumur, 1630.

CHAP. I.—Qui est celui qui parle sans langue, et comme il l'a perduë.

En matiere d'histoire bien recherchée la personne qui en est la suiect et qu'on desire faire cognoistre y doit estre tellement designée par sa naissance, son nom, son aage, sa condition, sa patrie, et sa constitution qu'il n'y ait rien à desirer pour le distinguer d'avec les autres. Or, cellui-cy, la merveille duquel oblige ma plume à tracer ces lignes, crayoñer son pourtrait, et d'en faire voir au jour le poncis en son plan naturel, est un garçon aagé de huit à neuf ans appellé Pierre Durand, fils d'André Durand et de Marguerite Salé, laboureurs du village de la Rangezière, parroisse Sainct-Georges près Mont-aigu en bas Poictou, lequel en l'aage de cinq à six ans tomba malade de la petite verrolle qui attaque presque tout le monde, et fait souvent des ravages estranges en quelques personnes, et principalement aux enfans et à la face, ou sa malignité exerce plus furieusement la rigueur de sa tyrannie, ce qu'elle fit d'une telle sorte à l'endroit de cet enfant qu'il en perdit toute la langue par la gangrène et pourriture qui se mit en sa bouche, ainsi qu'elle a de coustume en telle maladie à faute d'y prendre garde et d'y apporter le secours nécessaire d'assez bonne heure, à cause de la malignité du venin puissant qui l'accompagne, et de la nature chaude, humide et molle de ceste partie infectée, de façon qu'il la cracha par morceaux, sans qu'il luy en soit resté aucune apparence. Ce que neant moins ne l'empesche à present que fort peu de faire les cinq fonctions ordinaires qu'on attribuë à ceste partie qu'il a ainsi perduë, qui sont comme nous dirons ailleurs, de Parler, de Gouster, de Cracher, d'Amasser dans la bouche et d'Avaler ce qui s'y rencontre, pourceque cette bouche élanguée a nouvellement acquis une autre conformation fort propre à ces cinq actions, afin de subvenir aux necessitez de la langue, par la prudence admirable de la nature qui ne manque jamais aux occasions de se faire voir comme une mère à ses enfans.

The style of the work may be inferred from the above specimen of the first chapter. The subsequent chapters have the following titles:

CHAP. II. Quelle est la conformation de la bouche qui parle sans langue.

CHAP. III. De la construction naturelle et de l'usage ordinaire de la langue en l'homme.

CHAP. IV. Qu'il n'y a point d'apparence que la langue perdue se puisse s'engendrer.

CHAP. V. Pourquoy ceux qui ont perdu une partie notable du bout de la langue ne parlent plus sans artifice.

CHAP. VI. Comment c'est qu'on peut parler naturellement sans langue et sans artifice, et que cet enfant parle ainsi.

CHAP. VII. D'où vient qu'on peut sans l'aide de la langue, gouster, et cracher ce qui est dans la bouche.

APPENDIX E.

THE ORIGINAL STATEMENT OF DR. TULP RESPECTING JOANNES THE DUMB.

From '*Nicolai Tulpii Observationes Medicæ.*'
Amstelredami, 1652.

Lib. I.   Caput XLI.   Mutus loquens.

JOANNES (cui muti cognomen imposuit infortunium) petiturus Italiam incidit in pyratas Turcicos, quorum religioni nomen dare quum renueret, adnixi fuêre homines feroces linguam propterea radicitus ipsi evellere: sed per plagam, ex vulgi sententiâ, sub mento inflictam. Verum eâ credulitate minus ex voto ipsis succedente, detruncârunt ipsi deinceps totam illam partem, quæ lingua homini volubilis est, eâque ademptâ privârunt hominem omni voce.

Quâ tres amplius annos ubi caruisset, evenit forte ut intempestâ nocte admodum percelleretur ab inopinato fulgure: cujus pernicissimum lumen, cœlitus emissum perstrinxit usque eo pavidum ipsius animum, ut inde ipsi non secus ac olim Crœsi filio dissolveretur violenter tenax illud vinculum quod ipsum sermonis usu adhuc privaverat.

Quem tamen ubi vidit sibi restitutam, vix credidit sibi ipsi loquenti, nedum ipsi alii. Commovit quippe hæc inexspectata ipsius vox usque eo totam familiam, ut inde pro.

tinus abortierit juvencula ipsi cohabitans. Quo rumore latius deinceps sese diffundente, ivimus et nos tandem Wesopum, modicum Hollandiæ oppidum : spectatum coram insolitam hujus rei novitatem, famâ certe suâ nequaquam inferiorem.

Qui enim integrum triennium obmutuerat ob mutilatam mediam linguæ partem, cum audivimus cum eodem vitio non tantum distinctè loquentem : sed etiam accuratè pronunciantem quascunque literas consonantes : quarum tamen enunciationem solius linguæ apici attribuunt sagaciores naturæ indagatores.

Sermo quippe non formatur sine motu, nec consonantes sine linguæ apice. Quatenus enim lingua volubilis, eatenus distinguit vocem in verba : et prout allidit, vel ad dentes, vel ad palatum, aut labia : pro eo creditur etiam eruditis discernere vocabula et modulari concinne sermonis sonum.

Ac proinde haud mirum, læsâ tam evidenter linguâ, genuino dearticulatæ vocis instrumento, læsam utique fuisse et ipsam vocem : sed eandem, post triennii obmutescentiam manente linguâ perinde mutilatâ, INTEGRE ipsi nihilominus rediisse, id sane excedit omnium eruditorum captum : potuit quippe non modo expeditè clamare (id enim et aliis integrum fuit, post abscissam, resolutam, vel ligatam linguam) sed distinxit quoque perspicuè vocem in vocabula, et elocutus fuit omnia admodum articulatè.

Sed ut explicem me clarius quo ad repagulum a fulgure disruptum, asseveravit mihi candidè, se protenus a fulgure percepisse majorem motum in musculis linguæ. Quasi sublato jam inæquali illo coalitu quem sub mento reliquerat vulnus ibidem a pyratis ruditer sanatum. Verum deglutitio (cui non minus quam elocutioni inservit lingua) mansit ipsi perinde impedita; adeo ut ingenuè conquestus sit, ne tantulum quidem alimenti, etiam tum temporis, transmittere gulam, nisi id in eam intruderet violento digitorum suorum adminiculo.

APPENDIX F.

REPORT OF M. JUSSIEU TO THE FRENCH ROYAL ACADEMY OF SCIENCES ON THE PORTUGUESE CASE.

Mémoires de l'Académie Royale des Sciences, Année 1718. *Sur la manière dont une ' Fille sans Langue' s'acquitte des fonctions qui dépendent de cet organe. Par M. de Jussieu,* 15 *Janv.* 1718.

J'ANNONÇAI au mois d'Avril dernier à M. l'Abbé Bignon et à l'Académie, dans une lettre que j'eus l'honneur de leur écrire de Lisbonne, l'Observation que j'y fis de la manière dont une Fille née sans Langue s'acquittoit de toutes les fonctions qui se font avec cet organe. Et comme le peu de loisir que j'avois alors ne me permettoit pas de donner une ample relation de toutes les circonstances de ce phénomène, je satisfais aujourd'hui à ma promesse.

La Fille dont il s'agit ici est née de parents pauvres dans un Village de l'Allenteïs, petite province de Portugal. Elle fut présentée à l'âge d'environ neuf ans à M. le Comte d'Ericeira, Seigneur aussi distingué par sa noblesse que par son amour pour les Lettres, lorsque dans la Guerre dernière il passoit dans cette Province en qualité de Commandant d'une partie des Troupes de sa Majesté Portugaise.

La nouveauté du fait ayant excité sa curiosité, pour la

satisfaire à loisir, il envoya cette Fille chez lui à Lisbonne, où je l'ai vûë deux fois consécutives, et l'ai examinée avec toute l'attention qu'il m'a été possible.

Elle avait alors environ quinze ans, et assés de raison pour répondre à toutes les interrogations que je lui fis touchant son état et sur la manière avec laquelle elle suppléoit au defaut de cette partie.

Le soir à la faveur d'une bougie, et le lendemain au grand jour je lui fis ouvrir la Bouche, dans laquelle, au lieu de cet espace que la Langue y occupe ordinairement, je ne remarquai qu'une petite éminence en forme de Mammelon, qui s'élevoit d'environ trois à quatre lignes de hauteur du milieu de la Bouche. Cette éminence m'auroit été presque imperceptible si je ne me fusse assuré par le toucher de ce qui paroissoit à peine à la vûë. Je sentis par la pression du doigt une espèce de mouvement de contraction et de dilatation qui me fit connoître que, quoique l'organe de la Langue parût manquer néantmoins les muscles qui la forment, et qui sont destinés pour son mouvement s'y trouvoient, puisque je n'ai vû aucun vuide sous le menton, et que je ne pouvois attribuer qu'à ces muscles le mouvement alternatif de cette éminence.

M'étant rendu certain de la disposition de toutes les parties de la Bouche par rapport au défaut de la Langue, je fis un examen particulier de la manière dont cette Fille s'acquittoit des cinq fonctions ordinaires auxquelles cette partie est destinée.

La première, qui est le *parler*, se fait chés elle si distinctement et si aisément que l'on ne pourroit croire que l'organe de la parole lui manque, si l'on n'en étoit prévenu. Car elle prononça devant moi, non-seulement toutes les Lettres de l'Alphabet, et plusieurs syllabes séparément, mais même une suite de mots faisant un raisonnement entier. Je remarquai néantmoins que parmi les consonnes il y en a certaines qu'elle prononce plus difficilement que d'autres, comme le C. F. G. L. N. R. S. T. X. et le Z, et que lorsqu'elle est obligée de les prononcer lentement ou séparément, la peine qu'elle prend pour les faire sonner, se manifeste par une inflexion de tête dans laquelle elle retire son menton vers le Gosier ou Larynx comme pour l'élever et en le pressant l'approcher des Dents et le mettre à leur niveau.

La seconde fonction de la Langue, qui est celle du goûter, se fait aussi chés elle presque avec le même discernement de la qualité des saveurs que nous pourrions le faire, puisque j'appris d'elle même qu'elle trouvoit une douceur agréable dans les confitures sèches que l'on lui présentoit.

La mastication me parut lui être plus difficile à exécuter, car, cette petite éminence que j'ai remarquée qu'elle a au milieu de la partie inférieure de sa Bouche n'ayant pas une étenduë suffisante pour porter et repousser entre les deux Mâchoires les aliments solides autant de fois qu'il est nécessaire jusqu'à ce qu'ils soient réduits en pâte, elle employe à cette fonction le Mouvement de la Mâchoire inférieure qu'elle avance ou qu'elle éloigne du côte des Dents molaires ou Machelières de la supérieure, sous lesquelles se trouve le morceau d'aliment qu'elle veut briser ; elle fait même quelquefois servir un de ses doigts à cet usage.

Mais il n'y a point de fonction à quoi ils lui servent plus efficacement dans certaines occasions que pour la déglutition des solides, à laquelle la Langue est si nécessaire pour les pousser droit au Pharynx, lorsqu'ils ont été préparés par la mastication, et que comme une espèce de cuillier, elle en a recüeilli jusqu'à la moindre parcelle de tous les côtés de la Bouche. C'est principalement lorsque les parties d'aliment qui lui sont présentées se trouvent être ou plus difficiles, et par conséquent plus longtemps à être mouluës, ou qu'ayant besoin d'une plus grande quantité de salive pour être détrempées, les glandes salivaires de sa Bouche déjà épuisées par une longue mastication ne sont plus suffisantes pour lui fournir assés d'humide pour se couler aisément et d'elle-même à l'entrée de l'œsophage.

Pour ce qui est des boissons, elle ne diffère dans la manière de les avaler que par la précaution qu'elle prend de ne s'en pas verser tout à la fois une si grande quantité que les autres personnes, et d'incliner un peu sa tête en avant pour les avaler, afin qu'en diminuant la pente qu'elles auroient, si elle tenoit la tête droite, elle puisse moins s'en engorger. L'éminence même qu'elle a au milieu de la Bouche à la place de la Langue ne lui est pas inutile pour garantir le Larynx d'un trop grand abord de boisson par le petit obstacle qui l'oblige à se diviser, et à prendre la route ordinaire des liquides.

A l'égard de l'action de *cracher*, que l'on ne peut pas dire dépendre absolument de la Langue, mais à laquelle elle sert néanmoins si considérablement, qu'elle ne peut ordinairement s'exécuter sans son ministère, soit par le ramas qu'elle fait de la sérosité qui s'est séparée des glandes de la Bouche, soit par la disposition dans laquelle elle met la salive qu'elle a ramassée, ou la matière pituiteuse rejettée par le Poumon, pour qu'elles puissent facilement être poussées fort loin hors de la Bouche par une violente expiration ; à l'égard, dis-je, de cette action, il est vrai que la petite éminence est très-incapable de faire dans la Bouche le ramas de la Salive, et encore moins de la porter sur les Lèvres, mais à son défaut la partie inférieure de la Bouche remplie par les muscles moteurs de la petite éminence s'élevant presqu'au niveau des Dents de la Mâchoire inférieure, et les muscles buccinateurs s'approchant de deux Mâchoires, en expriment la sérosité et la conduisent jusqu'au Sphincter des Lèvres, d'où l'air qu'elle pousse avec impétuosité du Larynx lui sert comme de véhicule pour expulser cette salive, qui plus elle est épaisse, plus elle a de facilité à être jettée loin.

Je ne donne point cette relation comme un fait nouveau puisqu'il y a près de quatre-vingt ans qu'un nommé Roland, Chirurgien à Saumur, y a fait une observation semblable décrite dans un petit Traité, intitulé *Aglossostomographie*, ou Description d'une Bouche sans Langue, laquelle parloit et faisoit comme celle de cette Fille, toutes les autres Fonctions dépendantes de cet organe. La seule différence qui se trouve entre les deux sujets est que celui dont parle ce Chirurgien étoit un garçon de huit à neuf ans, qui par une gangrène causée par des ulcères survenues dans la petite vérole avoit perdu la Langue, au lieu que la Fille dont il s'agit ici est venuë au monde sans en avoir. Une circonstance même curieuse par rapport à son éducation est que ne pouvant, dans le temps que sa mère l'allaitoit, tirer comme font les autres enfans le lait par la suction à laquelle la Langue est si nécessaire pour le ramasser, et lui donner la direction vers le gosier, sa mère qui s'apperçut de la difficulté avec laquelle elle la têtoit, ne pouvoit lui communiquer son lait que par la pression de la mammelle dont cette Fille serroit le bout avec ses Lèvres.

La petite éminence que j'ai aussi remarquée comme singulière au milieu de la Bouche de cette Fille, fait une autre différence entre ce sujet et celui qui est cité par Roland, dont le petit Traité et l'Observation m'étoient alors inconnus, en ce que cette espèce de Mammelon qu'il dit qui restoit vers la base de la Langue emportée, était fourchuë et fort apparente, au lieu que celui de la Fille, dont je parle, est arrondi et n'est que très-peu sensible.

A l'égard des Dents de la Mâchoire inférieure, elles ne sont pas dans cette Fille à double rang, ni inclinées en dedans de la Bouche, comme dans le Garçon dont parle ce Chirurgien ; circonstance encore remarquable.

Si dans le nombre de cinq fonctions ordinaires de la Langue auxquelles j'ai remarqué que cette Fille suppléoit, il y en a quelqu'une de plus digne que les autres de nos observations, c'est sans doute celle de *parler*, surtout depuis que nous sommes assurés par les sçavantes recherches de M. Dodart que la Glotte est l'organe de la voix, et que les sons différemment modifiés dans la Bouche forment la parole.

Cette singularité d'une Bouche qui parle sans Langue doit donc servir à nous persuader qu'on ne peut pas conclure que la Langue soit un organe essentiel à la parole, puisqu'il y en a d'autres dans la Bouche qui concourent à cet usage, et d'autres qui suppléent à cette partie.

La Luette, les conduits du Nés, le Palais, les Dents et les Lèvres y ont tant de part, que des Nations entières se font distinguer dans leur manière de parler par l'usage dominant de quelques-unes de ces parties.

Pour ce qui est de celles qui peuvent suppléer au défaut de la Langue, je n'en ai remarqué aucune plus capable de remplir cette fonction que les muscles qui l'auroient fait agir si elle y eût été toute entière, mais principalement les Génioglosses, qui prennent leur origine de la partie interne du Menton, et viennent s'insérer presque vers la base de la Langue. Ce sont ces muscles, qui conjointement avec les Géniohyoidiens et les Milohyoidiens, tirant à eux l'os hyoïde du côté du Menton paroissent élever le Larynx et le rapprocher des Dents, en sorte que l'espace qui seroit entre les deux parties se trouvant diminué par cette contraction, la voix à la sortie du Larynx est beaucoup moins brisée qu'elle ne le seroit si la cavité de la Bouche étoit plus grande.

Et comme dans cette action ces muscles se gonflent, et acquièrent en se racourcissant un volume qui s'élève jusqu'au niveau des Dents, d'autant plus aisément qu'ils n'ont dans la Bouche aucun obstacle qui les empêche, ils semblent tenir lieu de cette rigole artificielle qui depuis le Larynx jusqu'aux Lèvres est formée par la concavité que prend la Langue pour porter la voix avec moins d'interruption au dehors de la Bouche.

Il y a même apparence que dès la plus tendre enfance de cette Fille, la nature avoit suppléé au défaut de sa Langue pour la suction des mammelles de sa mère, par le moyen de l'élévation de ces muscles sur lesquels le lait exprimé par les Lèvres tomboit, et étoit conduit directement au Pharynx le long de la rigole que forment ensemble ces deux muscles.

L'usage de cette rigole pour la suction a passé insensiblement à celui que je viens de lui marquer pour la parole, et s'est tellement fortifié chez elle par la coûtume avec l'âge, qu'on peut dire qu'elle fait à présent une partie des fonctions de la Langue.

La nécessité de cette espèce de rigole faisant en quelque manière l'office d'un porte-voix, ne peut être révoqué en doute, lorsqu'on observera que par son défaut causé, soit par une paralysie sur la Langue, soit par une tumeur ou inflammation à son extrémité, ou comme il arrive quelquefois chez les vérolés, par les brides qui la lient à l'intérieur des Mâchoires, lors, dis-je, qu'on observera que par quelques-uns de ces accidens on ne sçauroit plus entendre que des sons désagréables tels qu'ils sortent du Gosier, et par conséquent mal articulés.

La facilité avec laquelle cet enfant mutilé de la Langue, dont parle Ambroise Paré, s'exprimoit nettement, en approchant le bord d'un écüelle du tronçon de ce qui lui restoit de cette partie, est une preuve de besoin de la mechanique de cette rigole, et il y a lieu de croire que cet habile Chirurgien ne manqua pas de s'en appercevoir, si l'on en juge par l'instrument cavé en forme de goutière qu'il fit faire pour, en l'appliquant sur le moignon de la Langue à ceux qu'il verroit dans la suite mutilés de cette partie, suppléer au défaut de cette rigole.

J'ai dit que j'avois remarqué que lorsque la Fille dont il

s'agit vouloit prononcer lentement des mots composés de certaines consonnes, elle ne le pouvoit faire sans une inflexion de tête, dans laquelle elle retiroit son menton vers son Gosier comme pour l'élever, et en le pressant, l'approcher, et le mettre au niveau des Dents ; et cette observation sert à faire voir que la Langue n'est pas la seule partie qui agisse dans le parler, mais que les mouvemens du Larynx, de la Luette, du Menton, des Joües et des Lèvres y contribuoient aussi, tellement que leurs concours menagés sont capables de suppléer à la Langue même. Ce n'est que par le mouvement artificiel de quelques-unes de ces parties, qu'Amman a osé entreprendre de faire parlé les Muets dans le Traité qu'il a fait de la parole, puisque son art ne consiste qu'à leur faire sentir avec la main le mouvement du Gosier, du Menton, et des Lèvres de ceux qui leur parlent, et à les leur faire imiter en même temps en les aidant pour cela de la main.

Quelqu'un dans le doute où il seroit de la possibilité de parler sans Langue, pourroit s'imaginer que celle de cette Fille ne lui manquoit pas, mais que par un accident naturel elle auroit été colée à la partie inférieure et latérale de sa Bouche. Cependant il est aisé de lever ce doute par l'inspection de la Bouche ouverte, d'où non-seulement la capacité paroît plus grande, mais au fond de laquelle on apperçoit même sans peine la Luette presque du double plus longue et un peu plus grosse qu'à l'ordinaire, qui s'étendant jusqu'à l'Epiglotte, forme au fond du Gosier deux ouvertures égales et arrondies, au lieu d'une, qui quoique seule et pourtant beaucoup plus grande que les deux ensemble, ne paroît dans les autres sujets qu'en pressant la base de la Langue.

Cette disposition de la Luette, l'augmentation de son volume, et la diminution de l'ouverture du fond du Gosier produisent dans cette Fille beaucoup de facilité à prononcer les Lettres nasales par la liberté qu'a la voix de passer par les canaux du Nés. Il y a même lieu de croire que les sons qui sortent du Gosier de cette Fille n'auroient pu être que désagréables sans le petit obstacle que cette Luette allongée leur présente, lequel sert à leur donner une espèce de modulation.

Enfin si j'ai rapporté dans cette histoire quelques circonstances qui semblent la rendre conforme à celle du Chirurgien de Saumur, bien loin de les supprimer, j'ai crû au contraire qu'après les avoir exactement observées moi-même sur le sujet, je ne devois en oublier aucune pour que la possibilité d'un fait qui paroissoit extraordinaire demeurât plus avérée, et que l'on s'assurât de plus en plus que les parties renfermées dans la Bouche sont si nécessaires à l'action de parler, qu'elles peuvent dans cette fonction suppléer au défaut de la Langue.

APPENDIX G.

DR. NEWMAN ON ROMAN CATHOLIC MIRACLES.

Extract from Dr. Newman's 'Lectures on the Present Position of Catholics in England.' London, 1851: p. 298.

"I WILL avow distinctly that, putting out of the question the hypothesis of unknown laws of nature (which is an evasion from the force of any proof), I think it impossible to withstand the evidence which is brought for the liquefaction of the blood of St. Januarius at Naples, and for the motion of the eyes of the pictures of the Madonna in the Roman States. I see no reason to doubt the material of the Lombard Crown at Monza, and I do not see why the Holy Coat at Treves may not have been what it professes to be. I firmly believe that portions of the True Cross are at Rome, and elsewhere, that the Crib of Bethlehem is at Rome, and the bodies of St. Peter and St. Paul also. I believe that at Rome too lies St. Stephen, that St. Matthew lies at Salerno, and St. Andrew at Amalfi. I firmly believe that the relics of the saints are doing innumerable miracles and graces daily, and that it needs only for a Catholic to shew devotion to any saint in order to receive special benefit from his intercession. I firmly believe that saints in their lifetime have before now raised the dead to life, crossed the sea without vessels, multiplied grain and bread, cured incurable diseases, and stopped the operation of the laws of the universe in a multitude of ways."

Protestants are for the most part unacquainted with the evidence for many of the miracles mentioned in this passage. They know, however, something of the liquefaction of the blood of St. Januarius. The evidence for this miracle has received an unexpected honour in being pronounced irresistible by Dr. Newman. Yet it seems to break down on the threshold in this respect, that the red matter, called by courtesy the blood of St. Januarius, has never been proved to be blood at all, much less to be the blood of the saint with that name, who was beheaded in the beginning of the 4th century. The red matter has never been analysed by a chemist, and it is impossible by looking at it through the glass of the vial which contains it to know that it is blood. And considering the number of persons who in the course of centuries have had access to the red matter, historical evidence that it is the blood of St. Januarius cannot be regarded as trustworthy.

The miracles in Dr. Newman's list, for which it would be most interesting to know the evidence, are those involved in his belief that Saints in their lifetime "have crossed the sea without vessels," before the invention of balloons. Such seeming suspensions of the law of gravitation would be very impressive; and it would be easy to imagine such evidence for them as would exclude the supposition of art and contrivance. In reference to some of the other miracles, such, for example, as the motion of the eyes of the pictures of the Madonna in the Roman States, it would be difficult to disprove the existence of delusions, or of pious frauds.

APPENDIX H.

MIRACLES SPECIFIED BY DR. NEWMAN.

The nine miracles specified by Dr. Newman are the following:—

1. The miracle connected with the Thundering Legion.
2. The change of water into oil by Narcissus, a Bishop of Jerusalem.
3. The change of the course of the Lycus by Gregory Thaumaturgus.
4. Appearance of the Cross to the Emperor Constantine.
5. Discovery of the Holy Cross by Helena, the mother of the Emperor Constantine.
6. The sudden death of Arius.
7. The fiery eruptions on the Emperor Julian's attempt to rebuild the Temple at Jerusalem.
8. Recovery of a Blind Man by touching the relics of Gervasius and Protasius.
9. Speech without Tongues on the African Confessors.

I propose now to pass in review all the alleged miracles in reference to direct evidence for them, and the reality of their miraculousness.

Of these nine miracles, the last has been sufficiently discussed in the text, and may be withdrawn from the list as not being really miraculous though attested by eye-witnesses.

And the first and the sixth may reasonably be permitted to share the same fate. Neither of them is attested by an eye-witness; but besides this they are open to the objection that they would not be necessarily miraculous, even if all the alleged facts connected with them were admitted to be true: Theologians might possibly venture to call them providential; but this would be foreign to the present discussion, which deals only with the miraculous. I use the word miracle in this volume in the sense assigned to it by Dr. Newman, as "an event inconsistent with the constitution of the physical world," and, with him, I speak of events as miraculous "which have no assignable second cause or antecedent, and which on that account are from the nature of the case, referred to the immediate agency[a] of the Deity." But with this use of language there is nothing necessarily miraculous either in the events connected with what is called the Thundering Legion,[b] or in the death of Arius. As to the first point, what may reasonably be admitted is that in a

---

[a] See pp. 6-7, of 'Two Essays on Scripture Miracles and on Ecclesiastical,' by John Henry Newman. London: Pickering, 1870.

[b] The miracle of the Thundering Legion is so called from a statement that there was a Legion of Christians in the Roman Army under Marcus Aurelius, and that the Legion received its name of Thundering (Legio Fulminatrix) from its prayers having been supposed to be the cause of a thunder storm which saved his army. It is certain, however, that there had been a Legion of the same name (probably so called from the devices on the shields of the infantry) in the reign of Trajan, and in the times of Augustus. The subject is exhaustively treated by Mr. Moyle (b. 1672, d. 1721) in "The Miracle of the Thundering Legion, examined in several letters between Mr. Moyle and Mr. K——." (Moyle's Works, vol. ii. 1726.) All the original authorities have been collected by Mr. Fynes Clinton in his 'Fasti Romani.'—Appendix, vol. ii. pp. 23-26; accompanied by some valuable remarks of his own.

summer campaign against the Quadi in 174, the Roman army under Marcus Aurelius, when their supplies of water had failed through drought or had been cut off by the enemy, were relieved by a violent thunder storm which supplied them with water, and is said, by its thunder and lightning, to have disordered the Quadi. Now a violent thunder storm, with partially destructive effects, is a common event in summer after many days of intense heat, and such a common event cannot be rendered miraculous by its having been incidentally beneficial to Marcus Aurelius, and by the fact that one of its many antecedents had been prayer offered up for rain by Christian soldiers in the Roman army. It is to be remembered, moreover, that Marcus Aurelius had persecuted Christians before his campaign against the Quadi; and he persecuted them after his deliverance; and his death, though injurious to the Roman empire, was a gain to Christianity. Again, in reference to the death of Arius, there is no reason whatever for regarding that event as miraculous. Socrates[e] in his 'Ecclesiastical History' has given a detailed description of the way in which Arius died; and Sir Henry Holland, who has carefully read the whole passage, authorizes me to state that from the description of the symptoms, brief though it is, he is convinced that it was a case of abdominal disease, probably of the liver and larger intestines, which terminated thus fatally; and that sufferers from such disease not unfrequently die under cir-

---

[e] Φόβος ἔκ τινος συνειδότος κατεῖχε τὸν Ἄρειον· σύν τε τῷ φόβῳ τῆς γαστρὸς ἐκινεῖτο χαύνωσις· ἐρομενός τε εἰ ἀφεδρών που πλησίον, μαθών τε εἶναι ὄπισθεν τῆς ἀγορᾶς Κωνσταντίνου ἐκεῖσε ἐβάδιζεν. Λαμβάνει οὖν λειποθυμία τὸν ἄνθρωπον· καὶ ἅμα τοῖς διαχωρήμασιν ἡ ἕδρα τότε παραυτίκα παρεκπίπτει, καὶ αἵματος πλῆθος ἐπηκολούθει, καὶ τὰ λεπτὰ τῶν ἐντέρων· συνέτρεχε δὲ αἷμα αὐτῷ σπληνί τε καὶ ἥπατι· αὐτίκα οὖν ἐτεθνήκει.—Socratis, 'Historia Ecclesiastica,' lib. i. c. 38.

cumstances precisely similar to those recorded of Arius. Sir Henry Holland further states his belief from certain expressions in the description that Arius must have been afflicted with the disease for some time previously, though the fact may have been unknown generally to either his friends or his enemies.

Of the six remaining miracles the two first now on the list, viz., No. 2 and No. 3, may be briefly dismissed, as not attested even by a contemporary. The change of water into oil by Narcissus,[a] Bishop of Jerusalem, depends solely on the statement of Eusebius, who did not write his history till a hundred years afterwards. And Eusebius relates the story in such a manner as to render it doubtful whether he himself believed in it. He begins by stating, "Many miracles are recorded of Narcissus by his countrymen, as they received the tradition handed down from their brethren. Among these they relate a wonderful event such as the following." And then he narrates the marvel, accompanied by "they say." Again the marvellous statement that Gregory Thaumaturgus changed the course of the river Lycus is not attested by a contemporary. This miracle depends on the authority of Gregory of Nyssa, who was not born until fifty years after the death of his namesake, the wonder-worker.

For three other miracles, viz., No. 4, No. 5, and No. 7, there is some contemporary evidence, but no direct testimony of an eye-witness. The appearance of the Cross to Constantine (No. 4) is merely mentioned by Eusebius in his 'Life of Constantine,' as having been related to him, under the sanction of an oath, by that Emperor. But Eusebius is wholly silent on the subject in his 'Ecclesiastical History;'

---

[a] Bishop Narcissus seems to have been somewhat eccentric. Eusebius says of him that having been foully slandered, he ran away from Jerusalem, and continued many years concealed in deserts and unfrequented districts. (Eusebius, 'Historia Ecclesiastica,' lib. vi. cap. 9.)

and as Dr. Newman candidly remarks, the statement of what Constantine had said was not published in Constantine's life-time, nor till twenty-six years after the time to which it refers. So also the supposed discovery (No. 5) of the Holy Cross by the aged Empress Helena in 326 is not attested by any eye-witness. Moreover, it is not mentioned by Eusebius either in his 'Ecclesiastical History' or in his 'Life of Constantine,' and the earliest notice of it is by Cyril of Jerusalem twenty-one years afterwards. Even then Cyril is silent as to circumstances of time and place, and does not attempt to explain how the cross was identified. The absence of ocular testimony on this vitally important point is rendered peculiarly unfortunate by remarkable discrepancies in subsequent statements. All those statements agree in the assertion of what would be probable in itself—viz., that the crosses of the two Malefactors were found with the Holy Cross: but they differ widely as to the manner in which the identity of the Holy Cross was ascertained. Both St. Ambrose and St. Chrysostom, who wrote on the subject towards the end of the fourth century, assert that the Holy Cross was known by the inscription which Pilate had attached to it, and Ambrose quotes the exact words, "Jesus Nazarenus, Rex Judæorum;" though he says nothing of the inscription in Hebrew and in Greek. Moreover, both writers are so free from any doubt as to identification by the inscription, that each regards this result as the reason why Pilate had insisted on affixing that inscription to the cross.[*] On the other hand, all the ecclesiastical writers of the following

---

[*] See Ambrose, 'De obitu Theodosii Oratio,' and Chrysostom, 'In Joannem Homilia,' 89. The words of Ambrose are, "Hoc est quod petentibus Judæis Pilatus respondit, Quod scripsi, scripsi; hoc est, non ea scripsi quæ vobis placerent, sed quæ ætas futura cognosceret. Non vobis scripsi, sed posteritati; propemodum dicens, Habeat Helena quæ legat, unde crucem Domini recognoscat."

century concur in ascribing the identification of the Holy Cross solely to a singular test adopted by Macarius, Bishop of Jerusalem. According to them, Macarius caused all the three crosses to be brought to a woman who was lying at the point of death; and he ascertained the Holy Cross by its efficacy in restoring her to health, while the two other crosses failed in making any impression on her disease. The statement of the historian Socrates on this point is as follows:—
"A woman of the land affected with a disease of long standing, was at the point of death. The Bishop therefore arranged that each of the crosses should be brought to the dying woman, in the belief that if she touched the precious Cross she would regain her strength. And he was not deceived in his hope. For when the two crosses which were not the right ones were brought to her the woman continued dying not a whit the less, but when the third and genuine cross was brought to her, she immediately regained her strength, and became of sound health."[f] The historians Sozomen and Theodoret give almost precisely the same account of the test employed by Macarius, except that both of them speak of the woman as a person of rank or distinction; and Sozomen adds that the Empress Helena was present on the occasion. Now it is unfortunate that there is no statement by an eye-witness to make us certain as to which of the two accounts respecting the identification of the Holy Cross is to be accepted as true. If Ambrose and Chrysostom were in the right, a question would immediately arise why the Empress Helena did not take the same precaution to preserve the inscription, which she took to preserve the Cross itself. Of the many thousand inscriptions which have come down to us from ancient times, not one could even distantly have vied in interest with that inscription by Pontius Pilate, which would have constituted her title deed

---

[f] Socrates, 1, 17; Sozomen, 2, 1; Theodoret, 1, 18.

to the genuineness of her discovery. If on the contrary Socrates, Sozomen, and Theodoret spoke the truth, unpleasant suspicions would unavoidably arise founded on the unusual method adopted by Bishop Macarius for ascertaining an historical fact. It might or might not be unjust to suspect that he was a party to any pious fraud himself; but, supposing that he acted throughout in perfect good faith, his intellectual condition must have been such as to have rendered him an easy victim to the pious frauds of others. In the absence of further details, it would be dangerous to believe that, two hundred and ninety years after the Crucifixion, the Holy Cross and the crosses of the two thieves were really discovered by the Empress Helena, while Macarius was Bishop of Jerusalem.

Similar remarks apply to the eruption of fire at Jerusalem (No. 7), when an attempt was made by the Emperor Julian's orders to rebuild the Temple there in 363, during the last six months of his life. An eruption of fire on that occasion is mentioned by at least four writers who were living at the time—viz., Gregory Nazianzen, Ammianus Marcellinus, Chrysostom, and Ambrose; but not one of them was an eye-witness. And it illustrates the importance of ocular testimony to find that the two writers first named, who alone of the four were in the full maturity of manhood in 363, differ very materially in their narration of what took place. Gregory Nazianzen, in an Oration which he composed the same year, speaks as follows of an event which he designates as "much noised abroad and not denied even by the atheists themselves." After mentioning that the Jews joined with alacrity in helping to rebuild the Temple, he continues thus:[e]—

"But being interrupted by a hurricane and an earthquake,

---

[e] I adopt Lardner's translation, as being compressed and substantially correct. Lardner's Works, vol. vii. p. 604, edition of 1829. Gregory Nazianzen, Or. iv. pp. 111-113.

they ran to a church not far off either to pray or for shelter—and there are some who say that the church would not admit them, and that though they found the doors open, they were presently shut again by an invisible power. However, it is said by all and universally believed, that as they were using their utmost efforts to get into the church, a flame issued out from it, which entirely destroyed and consumed some of them, and scorched and maimed others in their members, so that they were living monuments of the justice and vengeance of God upon sinners."

On the other hand, Ammianus Marcellinus in his history which he published about twenty years afterwards, tells the story in a different way. He speaks of the preparations for the work, and of Julian's having entrusted it to Alypius who had held a high office in Britain; and he then states as follows:[h]—

"While therefore Alypius was actively urging forward the work and the Governor of the Province was seconding him, terrific balls of fire repeatedly bursting forth near the foundations, rendered the place inaccessible to the workmen, who were repeatedly burnt. And in this way the element obstinately repelling them, the enterprise was dropt."

Chrysostom in four separate passages speaks of the fire as coming from the foundations, and thus accords with Ammianus. Ambrose uses a neutral expression, that the workmen were burnt with fire from God (divino igne flagrârant). Ultimately it will be found that everything depends on a balance of evidence between Gregory Nazianzen and Ammianus, and the result is unsatisfactory. Gregory, who

---

[h] Ammianus, lib. xxiii. cap. 1. The four passages in Chrysostom are collected and translated by Lardner, vol. vii. pp. 605–607.

wrote in the same year, was an earnest and fervent Christian, but he was credulous and was sometimes very rhetorical. Ammianus, who wrote many years afterwards, was undoubtedly an intelligent historian, but he was at the same time a superstitious polytheist, not likely to be scandalized by prodigies or supernatural events in any form of religion. One intelligent eye-witness would have enabled us to decide between them, or might have led us to the conclusion that both were in the wrong. At present it is unsafe to attempt an explanation of the phenomena while there is such uncertainty as to the facts.

There still remains behind one miracle, viz. No. 8, which as far as evidence is concerned, is of somewhat more importance than others, and shall be therefore treated at greater length. This is the supposed recovery of sight by a blind man, called Severus, on touching supposed relics of two martyrs named Gervasius and Protasius. And at first sight this case appears to be attested by an eye-witness. But when the miracle is scrutinized, it will be found that all which is really attested by an eye-witness is that a man came forward *who said* that he had been blind, and that he had recovered his sight. But there is a total failure of direct ocular testimony that the man ever had been really blind.

The alleged miracle took place at Milan in 386, when Valentinian the 2nd, a minor, was Emperor, and his mother Justina was acting in his name. Both Justina and Valentinian were Arians, while the population of Milan, with its Bishop Ambrose, was intensely Athanasian. The fervour of their zeal as Athanasians is shewn by the fact that when in 385 Justina had demanded the possession of one of the Churches for her own religious persuasion, and when the demand was resisted by Ambrose, the Milanese took part with their Bishop and ensured his triumph. Indeed the religious passions of the population became so excited that

Ambrose himself was appealed to by Justina to restore tranquillity.

While there was this opposition of feeling between the court and the people, Bishop Ambrose, under circumstances which it is unnecessary now to particularize, was believed to have discovered the bones of the two Martyrs already mentioned, whose name and place of burial had been forgotten. Milan had been previously barren of relics; the supposed discovery was hailed with delight by the population; and the public removal of the bones constituted a kind of religious festival. One incident of the proceedings was the supposed recovery of sight by Severus, which is asserted several times by Ambrose and Augustine, who were both present. All the facts which they say they saw themselves may be received as undisputed; and there only remains one single doubt in the history of Severus, viz. whether he had or had not been really blind.

The Arians at the time denied the reality of his blindness. To this denial Ambrose[1] opposed, 1st, the assertion of Severus himself, which in a disputed case of this kind would certainly be of trivial importance, and 2ndly, the statement that the man was known in Milan, having been by trade a butcher, that he had given up his business on account of his malady, and that in proof of his blindness he had appealed to many inhabitants from whom he had previously received sustentation. At this distance of time, it is impossible to ascertain the precise truth respecting Severus. Probably, even if a special Commission of Inquiry had been

---

[1] See *Sanctus Ambrosius*, Opera, vol. ii., Parisiis, 1690. In page 878, there is an important passage which begins with a statement of the denial of the Arians. " Negant cæcum illuminatum, sed ille non negat se sanatum. Ille dicit, Video, qui non videbam, &c., &c."

immediately issued on the subject, the evidence would have been hopelessly perplexing; for an intense spirit of religious partisanship is likely to have existed at Milan, as the result of the recent conflict between an Athanasian populace and an Arian Court. It is, however, possible to shew that the evidence appealed to by Bishop Ambrose does not amount to direct ocular testimony for the fact that Severus had ever been really blind. With this object it is proposed to shew that from time to time cases occur of feigned blindness, and that the detection of imposture in such cases is difficult even for medical men, unless they have paid very special attention to the diseases of the eye.

There is a disease of the eyes called "amaurosis," which causes partial or total blindness without altering their outward appearance. Amaurosis (from *amauros*, dim, or obscure) is defined by the late Dr. James Copland in his 'Dictionary of Practical Medicine,' as "Partial or total blindness from affection of the retina or the nerves, or of that part of the brain which is related to the organ of sight, whether arising primarily from functional disorder, congestion or any other change of those parts, or occurring from sympathy with other organs," or in other words, "Partial or total loss of sight from other causes than those which obstruct the passage of the rays of light to the bottom of the eye." This is the disease which occasioned the total blindness of Milton, who nevertheless in well-known lines speaks of his orbs as

"clear
"To outward view of blemish or of spot;"

and in one of his prose writings he says of them, that "so little do they betray any external appearance of injury that they are as unclouded and bright as the eyes of those who most distinctly see."[1] When the difficulty of detecting feigned blindness is spoken of by medical men, reference is expressly or tacitly made to this disease of amaurosis. For blindness from other causes, as for example, from a cataract in the eye, could not be feigned successfully, although a cataract has been produced factitiously in order to escape military service.

To show the difficulty, however, of detecting imposition in amaurosis, total, partial, or intermittent, I proceed to give extracts on this subject from the works of three medical writers, viz. Dr. Copland, Mr. Marshall, and Mr. Tyrrell. And it may be useful to place on record trustworthy information respecting feigned blindness, not only as bearing on the case of Severus, but likewise as a preservative against imposture at the present day.

(1.) Dr. James Copland (b. 1791, d. 1870), in the 'Dictionary of Practical Medicine' above referred to, which is received in the medical profession as a standard work, has a separate heading for "Feigning Disease." In his Article under this head, after mentioning that defects of sight are frequently feigned, he writes as follows respecting a disease of warm climates called *night* blindness.

"Night blindness, or intermittent blindness (hemeralopia, nyctalopia) is often simulated by sailors and soldiers serving in warm climates, where the affection is common, and it is detected with difficulty. The deception is practised in order to avoid night duty, and has been put a stop to by associating a blind man with one who can see, in the various works carried on during night, and when the sentries are doubled."

---

[1] See Fellowes's Translation in Bohn's edition o Milton's Prose Works, vol. i. p. 235. Milton says in the original Latin that his eyes are "ita extrinsecus illæsi, ita sine nube clari et lucidi, ut eorum qui acutissimum cernunt."—*Defensio Secunda pro Populo Anglicano.*

These remarks are likely to have been founded on Dr. Copland's personal knowledge—for at one period of his life he had considerable medical experience on the western coast of Africa. He is a witness as to the difficulty of detecting feigned blindness by night; and this prepares the way for what follows.

(2.) Mr. Henry Marshall (— d. 1851), the author of a special work published in 1839, 'On the Enlisting, Discharging, and Pensioning of Soldiers,' more generally calls attention to the difficulty of detecting feigned blindness. He had been a regimental surgeon more than twenty years, and was subsequently Deputy Inspector-General of Hospitals, and he had thus frequently to consider not only the genuine diseases and disabilities which disqualify soldiers from service, but likewise the devices occasionally resorted to by individual soldiers for simulating disease, in order to obtain a pension, or discharge from the army. One of those devices was the feigning blindness; and I am indebted to Professor Sharpey for pointing out to me the following passage on this subject in Mr. Marshall's work.[1]

"Blindness without any obvious cause is sometimes pretended by soldiers, and there is reason for supposing that some of them are acquainted with the means of simulating the symptoms of this affection by the agency of drugs. The use of snuff which has been moistened with a decoction of *Atropa Belladonna* has the effect of dilating the pupil of the eye corresponding with the nostril into which the snuff was introduced. When any doubt is entertained in cases of this alleged disability, they should be examined repeatedly, and at uncertain periods. It may also be useful to propose an operation on the eye. Should the sense of vision not be

---

[1] Marshall 'On the Enlisting, Discharging, and Pensioning of Soldiers.' Edinburgh, 1839, 8vo., p. 103.

lost, the sight of an instrument may make a man wince and blink, by which means it will be obvious that he is not blind. Simulators of amaurosis sometimes discipline themselves, so that by shutting the eyelids an eye may not appear to be sensible to light, or to the presence of a sham instrument. Dr. Fallot met with a Conscript who had prepared himself in this way, and who by the aid of belladonna had completely simulated the principal symptoms of amaurosis. Having suspicions that the disability was feigned, he placed one hand over the region of the heart, and with the other appeared as if he intended to pierce the eye with a sharp instrument. The head moved not, but the heart palpitated, which induced Dr. Fallot to give a decided opinion that the disability was feigned; and under the influence of surprise and shame, the man avowed that his conclusion was correct, and he was consequently found fit for service."

(3.) There is a still more important passage of the same kind, written by Mr. Tyrrell, in a work entitled 'A Practical Work on the Diseases of the Eye.' (*London*, 2 vols., 1840). Mr. Frederick Tyrrell (b. 1797, d. 1843), at the time of his death, was unsurpassed as an eminent oculist. He was Senior Surgeon to the Royal London Ophthalmic Hospital; Surgeon to St. Thomas's Hospital, and Professor of Anatomy and Surgery at the Royal College of Surgeons, in London. The passage in question was pointed out to me by Mr. Bowman, himself so conspicuous for his great knowledge and undisputed ability in this department of scientific practice.

"Amaurosis is a disease which is very often feigned; and much difficulty occurs, in some cases, in detecting the attempt at imposition. In all these instances, both eyes are said to be affected; though perhaps one is described as most defective, for the purpose intended by the feigner would rarely be answered, unless all useful vision were supposed to be lost. Further, the eyes have generally a perfectly healthy character in appearance, on the action of irides, and in the feel of the globes; unless the party be acquainted with the effect of belladonna, or some other of the narcotics, which produce a similar influence, and have employed some previously to produce a dilatation of the pupils; this much increases the difficulty of detecting the imposture. The classes of persons who feign in this way are children, and apprentices, to get relief from tasks or work; or the latter to get free from an employment they dislike; soldiers and sailors to obtain a remission of duty; members of benefit clubs or societies in which liberal assistance is afforded to sick members. Now and then, I see a case in which I cannot detect any reason for the attempt to impose."

Mr. Tyrrell then proceeds to state, "I shall first detail the most marked difference between these cases, and cases of actual disease, and afterwards the modes of detecting the feigned disease." Omitting what Mr. Tyrrell writes under the first head as not immediately to the purpose, I will transcribe nearly all which he has stated as to the modes of detecting the feigned disease, as this will show how comparatively easy it would be to impose upon an unprofessional observer.

"The detection of the assumed disease may very often be made in getting the history of the case (provided the patient be allowed to tell his own story, which I consider best in all cases at first); for he is rarely sufficiently conversant with the ordinary symptoms to make a correct case; he will, probably, describe symptoms which are incompatible with each other, or such as could not exist without other evidence, or some material errors may be detected by the well informed medical man; at all events, by this means we gain much to lull or increase our suspicions. After this, an accurate examination should be made of the eyes without and with the aid of belladonna to dilate the pupils; for unless the disease have been of long standing, or the belladonna, or other matter producing the same effect have been previously used, the pupils will dilate from the use of belladonna, further than apparent when first examined; this may then enable the medical man to judge whether the pupils have been acted upon by medical means or not to aid imposition."

"During the explanation of the patient, and the examination of the eyes, do not if possible excite his suspicions of your opinion of any attempt at imposition; but rather endeavour to obtain his confidence by a little well-timed pity, and agreement with his account—you may thus often disarm him, while otherwise by creating suspicion you alarm him, and he is constantly on his guard; if he be unprepared, the sudden approach of the finger, or any extraneous matter to the eye will cause a sudden blinking if there be not amaurosis; or you may observe that his eyes turn quickly to any one you may address; or if you attract his attention mentally he will perhaps unintentionally be induced to direct and fix his eyes upon your countenance, as a person in earnest conversation usually does."

"When suspicion is excited, or when the party is well upon his guard, it is sometimes very difficult to prove the existence of visual power; but I have seldom failed to do this satisfactorily by perseverance."

"I have succeeded immediately by the following means. During conversation, dropping some small object as a knife or pencil suddenly, which has been immediately picked up by the patient; pretending to see something in the room or out of the window (if near) of curious or unusual character, the patient has been unguarded for a moment, and his eyes have followed the direction I have pointed to; asking how the patient's dress became torn or soiled, his eyes have been immediately directed to the part mentioned or pointed to; and several other like expedients."

"In one case of a little girl which baffled me for two or three weeks, during which period she had been strictly watched, but nothing elicited—I was engaged in conversation with her about her medicines, which she had much abhorrence of; and after trying to persuade her to take them well, I said I would give her sixpence if she promised to do so; she assented, and I held out a halfpenny towards her which she directly said (without touching it) was not a sixpence; she had previously sat for hours together without moving, and would allow me to place my finger or other matter in contact with the cornea without flinching."

The minute directions in this passage for baffling imposition strikingly illustrate the difficulty of detecting feigned amaurosis. Perhaps, however, no direction given to others on this point is more significant than the fact recorded by Mr. Tyrrell, that he himself was once baffled by a little girl during two or three weeks, although his suspicions had been awakened, and she had been strictly watched. This shows how possible it may have been to impose permanently on some medical practitioners, who were free from suspicion, and who had not made diseases of the eye their special study. And, in confirmation, it may be proper to mention a circumstance related to me by Mr. Bowman, viz. that medical men themselves have brought to him patients as blind, whom on examination he has discovered to be merely feigning blindness, and to be in fact impostors.

On a review of the above-mentioned facts concerning feigned blindness, it seems evident that there is no ocular testimony on record that Severus was really blind. Hence the alleged miracle of his recovering his sight constitutes no exception to the statement that of the nine alleged miracles specified by Dr. Newman, not one save that which relates to the African Confessors, and which turns out to be no miracle at all, is attested throughout by an eye-witness.

In conclusion, in laying stress on ocular testimony, it is not meant to deny that, under certain conceivable circumstances, the evidence of an eye-witness might be less trustworthy than hearsay evidence. This is true as an abstract proposition, but it is very far indeed from being applicable to any one of the miracles now passed under review. And as a general rule, other things being equal, ocular testimony is undeniably superior to hearsay evidence. It is true that some persons are extremely inaccurate even in relating what they have seen; but it is equally true that very few persons relate correctly what they have merely heard from others. When direct evidence ends, inaccuracy, if it does not exist already, is almost certain to begin. This is so well understood in England, that the general principles of English law exclude mere hearsay evidence from Courts of Justice. Hence in reference to early Ecclesiastical miracles—of which the Church of Rome itself does not pretend to possess any inspired or specially authentic record—it seems not unreasonable to require the testimony of some one intelligent and impartial eye-witness to some one of them, as a minimum of evidence.

APPENDIX K.

TILLEMONT.

The learned and excellent Tillemont, whose accuracy Gibbon has praised as almost amounting to genius, may perhaps be regarded as a fair representative of the ideas of the Church of Rome respecting the punishment of heresy. It is interesting therefore to observe how, in mentioning[*] Ulphilas and the Arian Emperor Valens, he deals with the Barbarians who received Christianity in the Arian form. Having spoken of the great missionary Ulphilas as "an instrument of the wrath of God," Tillemont says of him that "one man drew into hell an infinite number of Northmen, who with him and after him embraced Arianism." And of Valens he says that the Goths defeated his Generals, cut in pieces his armies, ravaged his provinces, and in the following year, after a horrible carnage of the Roman Army, burnt Valens himself alive, "that his punishment might have some proportion, even in the eyes of men, to the everlasting fires in which his crime plunged so many miserable beings." Tillemont, therefore, evidently believed that all the barbarians who during more than two centuries professed

---

[*] Tillemont's 'Histoire Ecclésiastique,' vol. vi., pp. 608–609. Paris, 1701–1712.

Christianity according to the creed of Rimini are doomed by the Deity to suffer punishment eternally in hell.

It may be doubted whether many forms of superstition have presented to the human imagination an equally execrable conception of the Supreme Being. Bacon says,[a] "It were better to have no opinion of God at all, than such an opinion as is unworthy of him; for the one is unbelief, the other is contumely: and certainly superstition is the reproach of the Deity. Plutarch said well to that purpose. Surely, saith he, I had rather a great deal men should say there was no such man at all as Plutarch, than that they should say there was one Plutarch that would eat his children as soon as they were born, as the Poets speak of Saturn." Yet the immorality involved in a God's eating his own children is trivial in comparison with the persistent cruelty and immorality of a Being who could inflict everlasting torments on the Northern Barbarians for having professed the creed of Rimini during their existence on earth. The idea of such a Being seems mainly due to theologians of the fourth and fifth centuries, who, disputing on subjects beyond the reach of their faculties, became heated by the fumes of controversy, lost their temper, took to cursing and swearing at each other, and then formed a God after the image of their own passions.

---

[a] Bacon's 'Essays.' XVII. Of Superstition.

APPENDIX L.

EDICT OF HONORIUS. A.D. 414.[*]

IMPERATORES HONORIUS ET THEODOSIUS JULIANO PROCURATORI AFRICÆ.

DONATISTAS atque hæreticos, quos patientia Clementiæ Nostræ nunc usque servavit, competenti constituimus auctoritate percelli. 1. Quatenus evidenti præceptione se agnoscant et *Intestabiles*, et nullam potestatem alicujus ineundi habere, sed perpetuâ inustos infamiâ cætibus·honestis et a conventu publico segregandos. 2. Ea vero loca, in quibus dira superstitio nunc usque servata est, Catholicæ venerabili Ecclesiæ socientur. 3. Ita . . . . ut Episcopi, Presbyteri, omnesque Antistites eorum, et Ministri, spoliati omnibus facultatibus, ad singulas quasque insulas adque Provincias exulandi gratiâ dirigantur. 4. Quisquis . . . . autem hos, fugientes propositam ultionem, *occultandi* causâ susceperit, sciat, et patrimonium suum fisci nostri conpendiis adgregandum, et se pœnam quæ his proposita est, subiturum. 5. Damna . . . . quoque patrimonii pœnasque pecuniarias evidenter imponimus Viris, *mulieribus*, personis singulis, et Dignitatibus, pro qualitate sui, quæ debeant inrogari. Igitur

---

[*] See the 'Codex Theodosianus Gothofredi.' Lipsiæ, 1743. Vol. iii. p. 194.

Edict of Honorius. A.D. 414.

Proconsulari, aut Vicariano, vel Comitivæ primi ordinis quisque fuerit honore succinctus, nisi ad observantiam Catholicam mentem propositumque converterit, ducentas argenti libras cogetur exsolvere fisci nostri utilitatibus adgregandas. Ac ne id solum putetur ad resecandam intentionem posse sufficere, quotiescumque ad communionem talem accessisse fuerit confutatus, totiens multam exigatur: et si quinquies eundem constiterit nec damnis ab errore revocari, tunc ad Nostram Clementiam referatur ut de solidâ ejus substantiâ ac de statu acerbius judicemus. Hujusmodi autem conditionibus etiam Honoratos reliquos obligamus: scilicet, ut Senator qui nullo munitus extrinsecus privilegio dignitatis inventus in grege Donatistarum centum libras solvat argenti: Sacerdotales eandem summam cogantur exsolvere: Decem primi Curiales quinquaginta libras argenti addicantur: reliqui Decuriones decem solvant libras argenti, quicumque in hæresi maluerint permanere. 6. Conductores .... autem domus nostræ, si hæc in prædiis Venerabilis substantiæ uti *permiserint* tantam pensionem pœnæ nomine cogantur inferre, quantum in conductione pensitare consuêrunt. Eadem quoque Emphyteutecarios auctoritas sacræ definitionis adstringet. 7. . . . Conductores vero privatorum, si permiserint in hisdem prædiis conventicula haberi, vel eorum patientiâ sacrum mysterium fuerit inquinatum, referetur per Judices ad scientiam dominorum, quorum intererit, si pœnam volunt sacræ jussionis evadere, aut certantes corrigere aut perseverantes commutare: ac tales prædiis suis præbere Rectores, qui divina præcepta custodiant. Quod si procurare neglexerint, hi quoque in pensiones quas accipere consuêrunt, prolatæ præceptionis auctorita mul(c)tentur, ut quod ad conpendia eorum pervenire poterat, sacro jungatur ærario. 8. . . . Officiales autem diversorum Judicum, si in hoc errore fuerint deprehensi, ad triginta librarum argenti illationem pœnæ nomine teneantur: ita ut si quinquies condemnati abstinere noluerint, coherciti verberibus exilio mancipentur. 9. *Servos* .... vero et *Colonos* cohercitio ab hujusmodi ausibus severissima vindicabit. Ac si Coloni verberibus coacti in proposito perduraverint, tunc tertiâ peculii sui parte mulctentur. 10. ... Adque omnia, quæ ex hujusmodi generibus hominum locisque colligi possunt, ad Largitiones Sacras ilico dirigantur.

Dat. xv. Kal. Jul. Rau. Constantio et Constante Coss.

APPENDIX M.

EDICT OF HUNERIC. A.D. 484.[p]

Edict of Huneric against the Catholics, called by him the Omoousians.

REX HUNERIX VANDALORUM ET ALANORUM UNIVERSIS
POPULIS NOSTRO REGNO SUBJECTIS.

TRIUMPHALIS majestatis et regiæ probatur esse virtutis, mala in auctores consilia retorquere. Quisquis enim aliquid pravitatis invenerit, sibi imputet quod incurrit. In quâ re nutum divini judicii clementia nostra secuta est, quod quibusque personis prout eorum facta meruerint, seu bona, seu forte talibus contraria, dum facit expendi, simul etiam provenit compensari. Itaque his provocantibus qui contra præceptionem inclytæ recordationis patris nostri, vel mansuetudinis nostræ crediderint esse renitendum, censuram severitatis assumimus. Auctoritatibus enim cunctis populis fecimus innotesci, ut in sortibus Vandalorum nullos conventus Omoousiani sacerdotes assumerent, nec aliquid mysteriorum quæ magis polluunt sibimet vindicarent: quod cum videremus esse neglectum, et plurimos esse repertos dicentes se

---

[p] See Victor Vitensis. Lib. iv.

integram fidei regulam retinere, postmodum universos constat fuisse commonitos, spatio temporis sibi prærogato mensium novem, novæque contentionis (si quid ad eorum proposita posset aptari) ut ad Kalendas Februarias anni octavi regni nostri, sine metu aliquo convenirent. Qui dum huc ad Carthaginensem confluerent civitatem post moram temporis præstituti, aliam quoque dilationem aliquantorum dierum dedisse cognoscimur. Et dum se conflictui paratos adstruerent, primo die a venerabilibus Episcopis eis videtur esse propositum, ut ὁμοούσιον, sicut moniti erant, ex divinis Scripturis propriè approbarent: aut certè quod a mille et quot excurrunt, Pontificibus de toto orbe in Ariminensi concilio, vel apud Seleuciam amputatum est, prædamnarent. Quod nequaquam facere voluerunt, universa ad seditionem per se concitato populo revocantes. Quin immo et secundâ die dum eis mandaremus ut de eâdem fide, sicuti propositum fuerat, responderent: hoc videntur assumpsisse ad temeritatem transactam, ut seditione et clamoribus omnia perturbantes, ad conflictum facerent minime perveniri.

Quibus provocantibus, statuimus ut eorum ecclesiæ clauderentur, hâc illis conditione præscriptâ, ut tamdiu essent clausæ quamdiu nollent ad conflictum propositum pervenire. Quod eâ obstinatione facere voluerunt quam pravis videntur assumpsisse consiliis. Adeo in hos est necessarium ac justissimum retorquere quod ipsarum legum continentiâ demonstratur, quas inductis secum in errorem imperatoribus diversorum temporum tunc contigit promulgari. Quarum illud videtur tenere conceptio, ut nulla exceptis institutiones suæ Antistitibus ecclesia pateret, nulli liceret alii aut convictus agere, aut exercere conventus: nec ecclesias aut in urbibus, aut in quibusdam parvissimis locis penitus obtinere neque construere; sed præsumpta fisci juribus jungerentur: sed etiam et eorum patrimonia, ecclesiis suæ fidei sociata suis Antistitibus provenirent, nec comeandi ad quæcunque loca

Edict of Huneric. A.D. 484.

talibus licentia pateret: sed extorres omnibus urbibus redderentur et locis: nec baptismatis haberent omnino aliquam facultatem, aut forte de religione disputandi; et nullam ordinandi haberent licentiam, sive episcopos, sive presbyteros, vel alios quos ad clerum pertinere contingeret, proposita severitate vindictæ, ut tam hi qui se paterentur hujusmodi honores accipere, quam etiam ipsi ordinatores denis libris auri singuli mulctarentur, eo adjecto ut nullus eis locus esset vel auditus supplicandi; sed etiam si qua specialia meruissent minimè prævalerent: et si in hâc pernicie perdurarent, de proprio solo ablati in exsilium sub persecutione idoneâ mitterentur. In populos quoque præfati Imperatores similiter sævientes, quod eis nec donandi libertas, nec testandi, aut capiendi, vel ab aliis relictum penitus jus esset; non fideicommissi nomine, non legati, non donationibus, aut relictione quæ mortis causæ appellatur, vel quolibet codicillo, aliisve forsan scripturis, ita ut etiam qui in suis palatiis militarent, condemnationi gravissimæ pro dignitatis merito facerent subjectos, ut omni honoris privilegio exspoliati infamiam incurrerent, et publico crimini hujusmodi personæ se cognoscerent esse subjectos; officialibus etiam judicum diversorum tricena argenti pondo pœna proposita: quam si quinque vicibus in errore perdurantibus contigisset inferre, tum demum tales convicti, atque subjugati verberibus, in exsilium mitterentur. Deinde codices universos sacerdotum, quos persequebantur, præceperant ignibus tradi. Quod de libris hujusmodi, quibus sibi dominis illius errorem persuasit iniquitas, præcipimus faciendum. Hæc enim, ut dictum est, pro singulis quibusque personis illi observanda præceperant, ut Illustres singulatim auri pondo quinquagena darent, spectabiles auri pondo quadragena, Senatores auri pondo tricena, populares auri pondo vicena, Sacerdotes auri pondo tricena, decuriones auri pondo quina: negotiatores auri pondi quina: plebeii auri pondo quina: circumcelliones argenti pondo dena. Et si qui forte in hâc pernicie permanerent, confiscatis omnibus rebus suis, exsilio mulctarentur. Ordines autem civitatum, sed et procuratores et conductores possessionum tali poenâ jubebantur affligere, ut si forte tales celare deligerent, et minimè publicassent, et retentos judicio non facerent præsentari, ipsi tenerentur ad poenam; conductoribus etiam regalium prædiorum hac mulctâ propositâ, ut quantum domui regiæ inferrent, tantum etiam fisco, poenæ nomine, cogerentur exsolvere. Id generaliter in omnibus conductoribus vel possessoribus qui in eâdem superstitione crediderint perdurandum, constituêrunt observari. De judicibus etiam qui huic rei instantissimè non imminebant, poenâ proscriptionis et sanguinis supplicio punirentur. Sed et de primatibus officiorum tres numero punirentur, aliis viginti librarum auri condemnatione mulctandis.

Quare his necesse est constitutionibus obligari Omoousianos omnes, quos hujusmodi malæ persuasionis constat tenuisse et tenere materiam. Quos ab omnibus supradictis abstinere decernimus, in prosecutionem venturis per ordines cunctarum urbium; sed etiam judices qui superioribus neglectis dira supplicia diversis non intulisse monstrantur. Omnes ergo supradictæ fidei ὁμοούσιον erroribus implicatos, quæ cuncto prædamnata est concilio tantorum numero sacerdotum, universis rebus prædictis, et contractibus præcipimus abstinere, quod nihil sibi noverint esse permissum; sed universos similis pœna maneat et adstringat, si ad veram religionem, quam veneramur et colimus, intra diem Kalendarum Juniarum anni octavi regni nostri conversi non fuerint. Diem autem præstitutum ideo pietas nostra constituit ut prædamnantibus errorem indulgentia non negetur, et obstinatos animos supplicia digna coerceant. Qui autem in eodem errore permanserint, seu domûs nostræ occupati militiâ, seu forsitan diversis titulis necessitatibusque præpositi pro gradibus suis descriptas superius mulctarum illationes cogantur excipere,

Edict of Huneric. A.D. 484.

nihil valituris quæ forsitan per subreptionem quemquam talium contigit promereri. In privatis etiam vel cujuscumque gradûs et loci personas hoc nostra promulgatio præcepit observandum, quod circa tales supradictis legibus videbatur expressum, ut pœnis congruis subderentur. Judices autem provinciarum quod statutum est negligentes exsequi superiori pœnâ, quæ talibus est præscripta, constituimus obligandos.

Veris autem majestatis divinæ cultoribus, id est sacerdotibus nostris, ecclesias universas, vel totius cleri nominis supradicti quibuscumque terris et regionibus constitutas, quæ, propitiâ divinitate, imperii nostri regimine possidentur, unà cum rebus quæ ad easdem pertinent, hoc decreto statuimus debere proficere; non dubitantes plus alimoniæ inopum proficere, quod sacrosanctis pontificibus justè collatum est. Hanc ergo legem, e fonte justitiæ profluentem, cunctis præcipimus innotescere, quatenus nullus sibi ignotum esse quod præceptum est, possit obtendere. Optamus vos bene valere.

Data sub die vi. Kalendas Martias, Carthagine.

INDEX.

A.

ÆNEAS OF GAZA on the African Confessors, 34, 36, 170
African Confessors, on the miracle of the, 5, 32; Victor Vitensis, 32; Gibbon, 34; Æneas of Gaza, 34, 36; Dr. Newman, 36, 42; Procopius of Cæsarea, 38; Emperor Justinian, 39; Count Marcellinus, 40; Victor, Bishop of Tonno, 41; Pope Gregory I. 41; Dr. Berriman, 68; Dr. Middleton, 72; Original Authorities, 169
Aglossostomography, or description of a mouth without a tongue, 52, 183
Agnus Dei—medium of divine manifestations and graces, 3
Alypius, 205
Amaurosis, defined, 208; difficulty of detecting imposition in, 209
Ambrose, St., an Italian by birth, 15; on the Holy Cross and the Empress Helena, 202, 203; on recovery of sight by a blind man, 206, 207, 208
Ammianus Marcellinus, 205, 206
Andrew, St., lies at Amalfi, 196, shone brightly in the dark, 4

Anthony, St., marvellous consequences have attended his invocation, 3
Arius, death of, 200
Augustine, St., an African by birth, 15; approved of the persecution of the Donatists, 20; letter to Count Marcellinus, and death, 23; quoted, 16
Authorities, original, for the history of the African Confessors, 169
Avidius Cassius, 16

B.

BACON on superstition as contumely, and the reproach of the Deity, 217
Beraudin, Gabriel, case of, 181
Berriman, Dr., on the African Confessors, 68
Bethlehem, the Crib of, is at Rome, 3; the fact firmly believed, 196
Boddington, Mr. Benjamin, 79, 83, 167
Boniface, Roman Governor of Africa, immediate success of the Vandals mainly owing to his disloyalty; bitterly repented of his treachery, 16

BOWMAN.

Bowman, Mr., 214
Brodie, Sir Benjamin, letter of, on the excision of the tongue, 108

C.

CECILIA, ST., axeman unable to sever her head from her body, 4
Chrysostom, St., 202, 203, 204, 205
Churchill, Colonel, 101, 103
Clarke, Mr. Fairlie, 48
Constantine, the Emperor, appearance of the Cross to, 201
Copland, Dr. James, 209
Crespin, Jean, account of French Protestant Martyrs, 180
Cross, the Holy, discovery of, by Empress Helena, 202
Cross, appearance of to Constantine, 201; discovery of the Holy Cross by the Empress Helena, 202-204
Cutting, Margaret, case of, 77; described in the 'Philosophical Transactions,' 78

D.

DICKSON, Mr. Joseph Ritchie, 114
Donatists, the, Schism from the African Catholics, 18; Analogy between, and the Scotch Free Church, 19; Persecution of, 20
Drelincourt, M., 88
Duncan, Dr. Marc, 51
Durand, Pierre, case of, 52, 183

E.

EDICT of Honorius, 218; of Huneric, 221
Ennius, memorable line of, 17
Ericeira, Conde da, 59
Eusebius, the Ecclesiastical Historian, sole authority for the

GREGORY.

statement that Bishop Narcissus changed water into oil, 201; mentions, in his life of Constantine, the appearance of the Cross to that Emperor, but is silent on the subject in his 'Ecclesiastical History,' *ibid.;* silent as to the discovery of the Holy Cross by the Empress Helena, 202

F.

FALLOT, Dr., 211
Faraday, Professor, letter of, on the case of Mr. Rawlings, 148
Faris, the Emir, case of, 100
Frances, St., saw her guardian angel, 4.
Francis, St., the cord of, is the medium of divine manifestations and graces, 3
French Protestant Martyrs, 180
Functions, the five ordinary, of the tongue — speaking, tasting, masticating, swallowing, spitting, 53, 62

G.

GENSERIC, invasion of Africa by, 15; persecution of the Catholics by, 23
Gervasius and Protasius, their bones supposed to have been discovered at Milan, 206; alleged miracle connected with them, 207
Gibbon, 5, 28, 34
Gregory I., Pope, on the African Confessors, 41, 173
Gregory Nazianzen, 204, 205, 206
Gregory of Nyssa, 201
Gregory Thaumaturgus, said to have miraculously changed the course of the river Lycus, 201

H.

HAMMOND, Mr., 80, 83, 167
Historia Persecutionis Vandalicæ,' by Victor Vitensis, 169
Homoousians, the, 27, 221, 224
Holland, Sir Henry, his statement respecting the disease of which Arius died, 200, 201
Honorius, Edict of, 218
Huneric, 24; persecution of the Catholics by, 24; Edict of, 26, 31, 221
Huxley, Prof., report of, on the case of Mr. Rawlings, 143

I.

ISIDORE, Archbishop of Seville, on the African Confessors, 71, 175

J.

JANUARIUS, ST., his blood liquefies at Naples, 3; impossible to withstand the evidence for its liquefaction, 9; the red matter so called has never been proved to be blood at all, 197
Jerusalem, fiery eruptions connected with the attempt to rebuild the Temple there, 204, 205, 206
Joannes the Dumb, case of, 54
Julian, the Emperor, ordered the Temple at Jerusalem to be rebuilt, 204
Jussieu, M. Antoine de, Report on the case of the Portuguese girl, 58, 60, 187
Justina, mother of Valentinian II., acted in his name when he was a minor, 206
Justinian, Emperor, on the African Confessors. 39, 89, 172

K.

KHISHT, a village between Abusheher and Shiraz, 99

L.

LYELL, Sir Charles, letter of, on the case of Mr. Rawlings, 142

M.

MACARIUS, Bishop of Jerusalem, singular test adopted by him to identify the Holy Cross, 203, 204
Madonna, impossible to withstand the evidence for the motion of her eyes in the Roman States, 196; in reference to such motion, difficult to disprove delusions or pious frauds, 197
Malcolm, Sir John, case attested by, 97
Mangin, Etienne, case of, 180
Marcellinus, Count, on the African Confessors, 40, 170. Another Count Marcellinus mentioned, 22, 25
Marcus Aurelius quoted Ennius in reference to enforcing discipline among the Legions in Syria, 17; his expedition against the Quadi, in A.D. 174, and his persecution of Christians, 200
Marshall, Mr. Henry, 210
Marshall, Mr. James Garth, 120
Martyrs, French Protestant, 180.
Matthew, St., lies at Salerno, 196
McNeill, Sir John, knew several persons in Persia who, although their tongues were cut out, could speak so as to trans-

MEHDEE.

act important business, 105; his letter on the subject, 107, 108

Mehdee Kooly Beg, case of, 116, 117

Middleton, Dr. Conyers, on the African Confessors, 49, 68, 72, 97

Milan, alleged miracle which took place at, 207; the populace Athanasian, the Court Arian, 208

Milman, Dean, letter of, on the case of Mr. Rawlings, 147

Milton, on cloistered virtue, 18; his blindness owing to Amaurosis, 208, 209

Miracles, Dr. Newman on, 2, 196: nine, specified by Dr. Newman, 198; definition of a miracle, 199

Mahommed Sadik, case of, 117, 119

Monza, the Iron Crown at, is formed out of a nail of the Cross, 3; no reason seen to doubt the material, 196

N.

NARCISSUS, Bishop of Jerusalem, said to have turned water into oil, 201; seems to have been somewhat eccentric, 201

Newman, Dr., 2, 4, 8, 9, 10, 11, 33, 36–44, 71, 75, 76; remarks on the evidence for the power of speech in the African Confessors, 176–179; belief in Roman Catholic miracles, 196, 197; nine miracles specified by, 198–215

Notcutt, Mr., 80, 83, 167

Nunneley, Mr. Thomas, report on the case of Mr. Rawlings, whose tongue he cut out, 122–138

RAYMOND.

O.

OLYBRIUS, 24

Owen, Prof., letter of, on the case of Mr. Rawlings, 148

P.

PAGET, Sir James, operated on the tongues of six patients, each of whom could talk quickly and intelligibly after the healing of their wounds, 158; in three cases, wherein he removed the tip of the tongue, the power of speech was not materially affected, 159

Paris, portions of the Crown of Thorns kept at, 3

Parsons, Dr. James, 78, 90

'Philosophical Transactions,' case of Margaret Cutting, in the, 77

Paul, St., was fed by ravens, 4; body of the apostle lies at Rome, 196

Peter, St., elicited a spring of water in the Mamertine, 4; his chair at Rome, 3; his body likewise, 196

Placidia, the Empress, ruled the West in the name of her son Valentinian III., 16, 24

Portuguese girl, case of the, 59, 187

Procopius of Cæsarea on the African Confessors, 38, 171

Protasius—*see* Gervasius

R.

RABBA ADAM, case of, 112

Raymond, St., was transported over the sea in his cloak, 4

RAWLINGS.

Rawlings, Mr. Robert, case of, 120
Roland, M., on the Saumur case, 51, 183
Roman greatness, cause of, and of weakness, 17

S.

SAUMUR case, the, 51, 183
Scholastica, Santa, gained by her prayers a pouring rain, 4
Scotchmore, Mr., a surgeon of Saxmundham, 81
Severus, his supposed recovery of sight, 206
Severus, the supposed blind man at Milan, 207
Sharpey, Professor, 210
Socrates, the ecclesiastical historian, his account of how Bishop Macarius identified the Holy Cross, 203, 204
Sozomen, 203, 204
Speech, modern cases of, with tongues amputated or wanting, 47; Pierre Durand, or the Saumur, 51; Joannes the Dumb, 54; the Portuguese girl, 58; Margaret Cutting, 77; Zâl Khan of Khisht, 97; the Emir Faris, 100; attested by Sir John McNeill, 105; attested by Dr. Wolff, 110; Rabba Adam, 112; Mehdee Kooly Beg, 116; Mohammed Sadik, 117; Mr. Rawlings, 120; attested by Prof. Syme, 150; attested by Sir James Paget, 157
Syme, Prof., 150
Syme, Prof., cut out the whole tongue of Mr. W——, after cutting through the under lip and sawing through the under jaw, 152; heard Mr. W—— speak in a loud clear voice, 154
Stephen, St., lies at Rome, 196.

W——.

T.

THEODORET, 203, 204.
'Theophrastus' of Æneas of Gaza, 170
Thundering Legion, miracle of the, and why so called, 199, 200.
Tillemont on the eternal punishment of Arians, 216
Tipasa, 30; emigration from, 31; mutilation of tongues at, 33
Tongue, five functions of, 62; not indispensable for purposes of speech, 162.
Tongues, modern cases of, amputated or wanting, *see* Speech, 47
Trèves, the Holy Coat is shown at, 3; no reason seen why it may not have been what it professes to be, 196.
Tulp, Dr. Nicholas, 54, 89, 185
Tyrrell, Mr. Fred., 211

V.

VALENTINIAN II., Emperor, a minor in A.D. 386, 206.
Valentinian III., Emperor, 16.
Vandal invasion of Africa, 15
Vegetius, on the disuse of defensive armour by the Roman infantry, 17.
Victor, Bishop of Tonno, on the African Confessors, 41, 173
Victor Vitensis on the African Confessors, 32, 169

W.

W——, Mr., of Manchester, case of, 151; while travelling in the

WILCOCKS.

Highlands, entered into conversation without betraying the loss of his tongue, 154

Wilcocks, Dr. Joseph, 58

Winifred, St., her well the source of wonders even in an unbelieving country, 3.

Wood, Mr., British Consul-General at Tunis, case attested by, 100; letter respecting three Emirs whose tongues had been mutilated, 103, 104

Wolff, Dr., the missionary, cases attested by, 110

ZENO.

X.

XAVIER, ST. FRANCIS, turned salt-water into fresh for five hundred travellers, 4.

Z.

ZÁL, Khan of Khisht, case of, 97

Zeno, the Emperor, 24

Printed in the United States
56401LVS00003B/74